Shauta, so
much for
your time
and support!

Love,

My Good Life

MY GOOD LIFE

One Woman's Quest to Raise Her
Special Needs Daughter

Eraina Ferguson

ELM HILL

A Division of
HarperCollins Christian Publishing

www.elmhillbooks.com

My Good Life

One Woman's Quest to Raise Her Special Needs Daughter

Published in Nashville, Tennessee, by Elm Hill, an imprint of Thomas Nelson. Elm Hill and Thomas Nelson are registered trademarks of HarperCollins Christian Publishing, Inc.

Elm Hill titles may be purchased in bulk for educational, business, fund-raising, or sales promotional use. For information, please e-mail SpecialMarkets@ ThomasNelson.com.

Scripture quotations are taken from the Holy Bible, New International Version', NIV'. Copyright © 1973, 1978, 1984, 2011 by Biblica, Inc.' Used by permission of Zondervan. All rights reserved worldwide. www.Zondervan.com. The "NIV" and "New International Version" are trademarks registered in the United States Patent and Trademark Office by Biblica, Inc.'

Library of Congress Cataloging-in-Publication Data

Library of Congress Control Number: 2019917718

ISBN 978-1-400328383 (Hardbound)
ISBN 978-1-400328390 (eBook)

TABLE OF CONTENTS

Prologue: Naked   *xiii*

1. Born Again   1

2. Good Family   13

3. Orphan   17

4. Concrete   27

5. Escape   31

6. Privileges   45

7. Good Love   61

8. Ever After   73

Epilogue: My Good Life Now   77

How to Use This Book

L ife is fluid. As I stood in front of a group of parents at the beginning of their journey, I was asked a question about how I got to the place of peace. They were describing the peace that resonated on my face while bike riding with Taylor on Martha's Vineyard. It was indeed a crossover point. In that moment of riding a bicycle and feeling a euphoric high of peace, love, and freedom, I vowed to return to that place often. To visit the mental state of peace that existed in that moment. Over the years I've revisited the photo, reminding myself that the good life is now—it is not a destination, but a mindset I must fight to return to daily.

That is how you should use this book. Read it, and at the end of each chapter, remember the good things that exist in your life from day to day. Are there things that you would like to change or see done differently? Change them. Set the standard and move toward the good. Build your good life one day at a time. Without lamenting, take the time to reflect on the possibilities that exist and move toward those possibilities.

For grandma, in all of my remembering,
I promise to remember well.

INTRODUCTION

G ood (adjective): Morally excellent; virtuous; righteous; satisfactory in quality, quantity, or degree; of high quality

*After looking up the definition, I realize that there is only one good thing: God.

And God said, "Let the water under the sky be gathered to one place, and let dry ground appear." And it was so. [10] God called the dry ground "land," and the gathered waters he called "seas." And God saw that it was good.

(GENESIS 1:9)

PROLOGUE

NAKED

I felt relieved as I drove my friend's 1994 Acura down Elm Street. I drove past Calhoun College and past the Yale Welcome Center. Right before I arrived at Church Street, my phone rang. I wondered who could be calling me. I knew it was not my boss; he had just blown me off. He was too busy to engage in a conversation about why I was unable to attend professional development training. Though I'd run into childcare issues in the past, the last few weeks had been challenging. I was at my wits end, trying to understand why I could not do this. I had done the impossible before. Seven years to the month, I completed the same type of teacher training at a program in New York. Back then I also had the odds stacked up against me, but I pulled out my scriptures and got on my knees and prayed. In June 2003, I moved to New York City with only a job, one thousand dollars, and a dream of a good life for me and my daughter Taylor. In the past I was equipped with the stamina to deal with this situation. I had nothing left to fight with. Thirty minutes earlier, I sat with my head in my hands and sobbed. My integrity would not allow me to keep this position. I must resign and move on because finding childcare had been impossible. Handing in the resignation letter felt like failure. Despite the circumstances, I was not worried about the future. I was grateful for a moment because I was able to breathe. I could take a sigh of relief that now I could move forward, knowing that I had not kept my employer at bay. I did everything I could to make this position work.

"Hello," I said.

"Hi Eraina, this is Rochelle from the dining facility at Yale."

"Hi how are you?" I asked. I had no idea why she was calling. I remember giving her my card months earlier as I did often, but I had no idea why she would be calling now. I listened, unaware of the difficult news that she would deliver.

"Eraina," she said, "please stay calm."

Stay calm, I thought, *why would I need to stay calm? What happened? Why was she calling?* A barrage of questions ran through my mind and my heart began to beat faster. I waited to hear what the difficult news would be.

She proceeded to tell me the devastating news. Taylor had run outside naked while with the babysitter. "I looked out the window and saw Taylor running down the driveway with no clothes on."

I pulled the car over as emotions flooded my body. I could not believe what I was hearing. After the initial wave of shock and disbelief flooded my body, anger and rage followed. I called the babysitter and yelled at her, asking how she could allow this to happen. Before I could spew more anger and rage, a calm voice took the phone.

"Hi Eraina, this is Anna Ramirez." *Anna Ramirez, the admissions counselor at Yale Divinity?* I wondered why the admissions director was calling me. She was the dean of admissions at the Divinity School. "As I drove by this morning, I saw Taylor and pulled over to help. Taylor is fine," she comforted. "Taylor is safe," she said, "just get here as soon as you can." She attempted to reassure me that everything would be okay. As I drove home, I felt relieved that someone else was there besides the babysitter.

It had been a challenging summer.

This was a huge blow. I had nowhere else to go. What would I do now? How could I care for this child with no job and no childcare? That is what this second Master's degree was about. It was supposed to place me in a position where I could excel in my academics and my career. I was so hopeful that I could finally have the career that I dreamed of and worked so hard for. As the tears streamed down my face, I was feeling low and prayed for something good to happen. As I pulled up to the front door, leaving my emergency hazards on, I tried to remain calm.

The babysitter had been in her office when Taylor ran outside. The challenging reality of raising a special-needs child is their limited understanding of danger. I used to be embarrassed by this story, worried that I would be judged. One lesson I learned at Yale Divinity was when one of my fellow classmates reminded me of the scripture when Jesus asked Adam, "Who told you that you were naked?" Sometimes our experiences are based on someone else's point of view instead of our own. Living in our truth is imperative for living the good life.

There are so many memories that stick with me. My memories are accompanied by visions, smells, and sounds that I cannot shake. I think memory is an important part of our makeup and invites us to move forward regarding our personalities. I compiled these memories to help me understand what happened during the twelve year span of raising Taylor on my own.

What happened in NYC, Boston, and New Haven to make up my personality and, most of all, the life that I worked so hard for?

My good life.

CHAPTER 1

BORN AGAIN

I gave birth to Taylor on October 2, 1999. I named her Taylor Gabriel Davis. I called her my tailor-made messenger. In the Bible, Gabriel was a messenger that brought the good news of Jesus' birth to Mary. I know that she was created for good news. I went into labor in the early morning hours. It was a Saturday morning when I first began feeling contractions. My mother arrived the previous week when the doctor informed me that I would give birth soon. I was excited and scared, not realizing how my life would be forever changed by the birth of this child. I first mistook my labor symptoms for indigestion. I gently woke up my mother, telling her that it felt as if I needed to belch or pass gas. She laughed and explained that I was probably in labor and that I should get as much sleep as possible. She predicted that my labor would be between twelve and seventeen hours. Though the pain eventually set in, there was not as much as I predicted there would be. I saw that as a good thing, a sign that perhaps this whole labor thing would not be difficult. I rested during my contractions and by 12:00 pm, the contractions started to become more intense and frequent. Thinking that it would still be a long time before I delivered, my mother rubbed my back while I took naps in between my contractions.

By 5:30 pm my contractions were closer together. It was hard to believe that I was about to give birth to a child that almost did not make it. Four months prior, I left my routine prenatal checkup numb with fear. The fear paralyzed me, and since I had a limited relationship with God for myself, despite being raised in a Pentecostal Church, I was unable to see past what the doctors informed me. They convinced me to schedule a two-day abortion at the University of Chicago Hospital. Several days before the procedure, I was overwhelmed with grief, and to hide my tears, I went into the bathroom. I pulled down the top of the toilet seat and sat with my head in my hands, sobbing uncontrollably. The pain and grief were physical now and had overtaken my entire body. I was distraught. Then I remembered what I learned as a youth in the Pentecostal Church. I got down on my knees and sang a song that I heard from the elders, "Yesssss Lord, Yes, Lord, Yes, Lord, Yeess Lord." I sang and sang and rocked and rocked back and forth, remembering the chorus of women who usually sang this song. I sang until I could no longer feel the pain. Until I forgot where I was. I sang until my whole body felt as if it were being held. Finally, the physical pain of the grief subsided. When I finally came to and realized where I was, I was in the fetal position on the floor, staring at a peach rug. I was interrupted by a knock at the bedroom door saying that Deila, my older sister, was on the phone. Deila had always been the forerunner in every aspect of growth.

She was the oldest and was first to attend college. She was the first to go away at a young age to serve as a congressional page. She was also more spiritually grounded than me. For most of my life, though I respected my mother, I feared my sister. She served as the third parent, which created an interesting dynamic in our relationship. Though I was emotionally drained, I was excited to speak to her. Her tone was enthusiastic, as if she had good news to tell me. She told me that she had been praying and that Taylor, as we already called her, was healthy. She told me not to abort. Instantly the pain lifted. Deila advised me to have the procedure that would test for chromosomal abnormalities. God heard my prayer on that bathroom floor. He guided me in the right direction. There is a little bit of good that is inside of all of us that leads us in the right direction. It creeps in at the most unsuspecting times and takes hold of every situation. It demands reciprocation and attention. It is pure and intentional.

We immediately called our ride and headed to the hospital. Though we arrived at 6:00 pm, everything went so fast. I was prepped in the delivery room and two pushes later at 6:45 pm, Taylor arrived.

Newborns are wrinkled and funny looking, but there was something so beautiful about Taylor. My best friend and I spent hours on the phone naming her months earlier. I called her Taylor while she was still in the womb. I often feel that I was too young to realize the huge impact this would have on my life. I did not realize how much responsibility I would have over the next decade. There would be changes and perils that I would experience. There would also be a host of sacrifices. I had no idea what I was in for. All I knew was that at that moment, I felt like the luckiest woman in the world. I was Taylor's mom and she was perfect, with no physical disabilities that I could see, and as far as I knew, she was a healthy baby girl. I had one day. One day to think of her as perfectly whole. I did not know as I slept and rested that in twenty-four hours, everything would change forever.

My default response to let her stay in the nursery was a result of the nurse's prompting. If I had not allowed her to spend that night away from me, I may not have discovered her disability. Me and my mom went to the nursery the next day to see her. As I slowly walked down the hall with my hair in a loose ponytail, I was excited to see her again. My child was healthy. A healthy baby girl. That is what the nurse told me months before after the amniocentesis. "You have a healthy baby girl." I looked through the window to the nursery and watch her from afar, as if I was trying not to alert her of my presence. She was so beautiful, and she had these large pink lips that looked as if they belonged to a two-year old. She was so beautiful. Her hair was black and soft, and I could not wait to hold her. She looked like her father. I could not help but reminisce on how we met.

I was immediately attracted to Kevin because of his good looks. He had the type of looks that were only seen on movie stars. He had clear caramel skin with a tint of a tan. Though he was sitting down, I could see that he was wearing khaki pants. The creases fell just right on his slender body. He wore a short sleeve oxford plaid shirt. His hair was cut low and chiseled almost to perfection. He looked intelligent, as if he used proper grammar and could hold interesting conversations. The habit of seeing the best in people would be a skill that I have mastered over the years. It was also my explanation for several failed relationships. He was what we referred to as a pretty boy. This would explain why his appearance was flawless. I would find out later that he was a barber. He was clean, neat, and beautiful. I was on another date when I met Kevin. During that time in my life, it was the norm to go out with a guy for a free meal. When the guy would ask for a form of payment later, I would casually decline.

I first noticed Kevin from across the room just as our check came. I bit my bottom lip to keep from breathing with my mouth open. I was in awe. I immediately started to plot on how I would get his number. My date sat conversing with the other couple that we came with. Without thinking, I made a quick suggestion, "Why don't you guys go pull the car around. We will wait for the check to come and pay the waitress." And then I could give the handsome guy my number. When my meal ticket left, I asked the waitress for a pen, wrote down my number, and walked over to the table. When my date was out of sight, I strolled over to his table and said, "My name is Eraina. You must call me." He did. We had long talks about nothing in my dorm room. I did what many women do, fantasized about who I wanted him to be while over-calculating his interest in me. Taylor was conceived the first time we were intimate.

A month later when I told him I was pregnant, he stopped calling all together. What I did not know when I strolled over to him in the restaurant that day was that he had a two-month old. I was nineteen and he was twenty. I can only imagine the fear he had knowing that he had a second child on the way. I was persistent though, and before I gave birth to Taylor, I visited him and eventually created a long-lasting relationship with his family that still exists. They make up in love and support what I craved from Kevin.

***

As I looked in the window admiring her, another parent walked into the nursery, causing the door to slam. Taylor's crib was near the door, but she did not jump. A noise so close in proximity should have startled her. I also noticed it because in this room, there were only five cribs. The other babies appeared to hear the noise but Taylor slept quietly, never moving an inch. *Interesting*, I thought. *I wonder why Taylor didn't jump?* I waited for another person to enter the room. I waited in vain for her to react to the door slam. She never did. Something was wrong. I dismissed any thoughts that I may have had regarding her hearing and went in to wheel her to my room. *She's probably just sleeping hard*, I thought. *I'm sure she is fine and hears perfectly*. I took her back to the room and held her close to me. I talked in her ear with a soft tone to see if she could hear, dismissing any negative thoughts I had about any hearing loss. I still speak to her just as I did in the hospital room, smiling and telling her how beautiful she is, mouthing to her that I love her.

I had no idea the doctors knew my secret. When we were given our discharge information, they expressed concern over her hearing. They provided me with the paperwork for a preliminary routine hearing screening. "Taylor failed the initial hearing screening Ms. Davis. Please bring her back next week and we will do another hearing screening."

"Thank you," I said. Masking the doubt in my face, I gave a phony smile, but on the inside, I knew that she was deaf. She could not hear. The previous day in the nursery confirmed it and their test was correct. I did bring her back the next week for the screening which she failed again. Tears rolled down my eyes as I left the hospital. No pity party though. For some reason I had a scary sense of optimism and closure. I rested in the reality of what would inevitably be a deaf diagnosis. I endured this experience alone, as I would do for so many years.

Before I arrived home, I decided that I would not have a prolonged period of grief over this new diagnosis. I felt as I have felt many times over the years that I needed to stay strong and accept this new reality sooner than later. My mother would be with us for another month before she returned to Florida, and I had only two weeks before I would return to school. I needed to learn how to take care of Taylor's basic needs and finish the program I was in. When I entered our first-floor apartment, I was determined to do just that. I needed to move forward and prepare for the reality that I would be left alone to raise this child with hearing loss. I carried her car seat in and unbundled my healthy baby girl, smiling at her after drying my tears. Before I knew it, Christmas had arrived, and the semester was over. We were headed on a plane to see my mother in Florida. Taylor was two months old and she was bundled in her Christmas-themed pajamas. It was a wonderful time.

The first couple months of her life were filled with the usual events of a newborn. We attended numerous doctor's appointments, including several failed hearing screenings. The doctor said it was too early to fit her for hearing aids and recommended we could explore other options. I always wondered how it was that we miss those good things in our lives. Many times, we are overcome by the bad events that life brings, and we miss the good. Even when it is a little bit of good, it is worth being recognized.

Despite her diagnosis, Taylor was a pleasant baby. For the first couple months, she played and interacted like a typical baby. When she failed to meet her milestones, we became concerned. She couldn't hold her head up, she could not sit up, and she took a long time to roll over. We enrolled her in early interventions, which is a program aimed at providing therapy for children with developmental delays to help them meet their milestones. During the assessment, she was diagnosed with global developmental delay. She had low muscle tone in her legs and could not stand or sit alone by her first birthday. However, she smiled constantly. She was a happy baby. Despite her limitations, I enjoyed feeding, playing, and loving her as if she were a typical child. Her speech, occupational, and physical therapies became a part of our daily routine. Overall, I was at peace with the diagnosis of her hearing loss. Some of my family members would clap their hands or enter the room yelling, and when she looked up, they proclaimed that she could hear. Yet it was the cues she learned over time that prompted her movement and not the fact that she could hear. I knew that it was painful for my family to see me go through those first few months.

I learned early on to not be emotional especially about my situation. My parent's move had a lot to do with this. Though my dad and stepmom lived less than an hour away, there was an interesting family dynamic that fostered independence and choice. It caused me to deal with my emotions on my own. It was a lonely feeling, but I made every effort I could to not get distracted by what other people did not do for us. I especially appreciated this family dynamic when it was time to leave Chicago. It was the easiest move I would make. I felt a sense of urgency to maintain focus.

When people asked me why and how I chose to embark on this spiraled journey of twists and turns, I realized that it all started with a decision. At twenty years old and a junior in college, I was already leading a challenging life. To some it looked difficult, but I found myself to be extremely blessed. I was a single mother of a hearing-impaired child and a full-time student. Growing up, I felt like I had four parents. I had two parents and two stepparents. I was accustomed to having everything I needed and some of what I wanted. I also had two loving grandmothers that lived within blocks of each other. I was unaware growing up that other children were leading difficult lives that presented hardships that I knew nothing of. My great aunt was an entrepreneur. Since moving to Chicago in the early sixties, she opened two small businesses. My grandparents lived a modest but comfortable life across the street from my then-Catholic elementary school. Life was good. The biggest uncertainties I had were whether my pleats in my uniform would be pressed to perfection or counting how many Peter Pan collar shirts I had to last for the week.

At the beginning of the school year, I always received at least two new pair of shoes, with my maroon knee-high socks, and a new book bag. Every year I insisted on purchasing a new book bag. I enjoyed my Catholic elementary school experience. After school, my stepdad Leroy would be waiting outside to collect us in the maroon conversion van with the televisions in the back. It was the late 1980s, long before the mini-van, yet these vans were state-of-the-art must-haves for families. It was a good life indeed, and I mistakenly assumed that everyone grew up with the same daily routine. My daughter's father would remind me years later that not everyone grew up the same.

I was a twenty-year-old single parent with no real means of income. One day I went to one of my favorite places in downtown Chicago oblivious to the issues that I faced. I was blessed with a dynamic childcare provider. She only charged me a mere fifty dollars a week. I was able to attend my classes during the day and eat lunch in downtown Chicago. After attending an afternoon class, I was able to stroll some evenings downtown on the Magnificent Mile. I loved window shopping in stores I could not quite afford. In my mind, one day I would be able to afford these places. I learned at an early age not to place limits on myself, specifically those set by others. Choosing silverware for my first apartment probably seemed like a bad idea.

Crate and Barrel was where yuppies and wannabes shopped for their post-wedding grown-up furniture. It was stocked with your traditional modern must-haves.

I was unaware that this was not the go-to spot for unwed single Black mothers, in their third year of college. I was totally oblivious to the fact that I most likely stood out. At the time, I had a young childlike appearance. I entered the store with my chin perched high as if I was on my way to register for my wedding. But the reality was that I was on my way to purchase silverware. I had wine taste with beer money. My palate was trained by my classy stepmother who gave me my first coach wallet at the age of fourteen. Silverware. I was there to buy silverware for my kitchen that was outfitted with a makeshift table and lawn chairs. I wanted the best silverware however, and Crate and Barrel was the place to get it. Though my great aunt possessed china cabinets full of china and silverware, I lacked the knowledge of how challenging it was to outfit a table. Since I could not afford to get a table setting for four, I decided to purchase a setting that would meet my needs. I purchased a setting for two and used the larger spoons.

Good Timing

There are so many opportunities for God to use us in our everyday lives, and it is often about His timing. I rushed around in anticipation for a specific event, and when it finally arrived, I was right on time. Have you ever been in traffic or minutes away from your destination and everyone is seemingly driving in slow motion? It was probably not your time to be there. My most vivid memory of involving good timing was during a drive to take Taylor to daycare when she was a baby. I lived downtown Chicago and her babysitter was in the Western suburbs.

One instance taught me a lot about timing and awakened me to the need for continual focus and urgency. One morning I woke up early and I quickly dressed Taylor and packed her into my 1999 Malibu. I was a junior at UIC and anxious to get to class on time. I rushed onto 290 West heading to the sitter. As we drove, I pulled into the center lane. I had a weird feeling that something wasn't right. In fact, it was moments later that I saw an accident occur right in front of me. However, before it happened in real time, I had the urge to slow down and pay attention to what was in front of me. A car swerved from the left lane, across my lane, hitting several cars in the far-right lane. As I slowed down, everyone in the back of me did as well.

By the time everything halted, there was wreckage in front, my car untouched in the middle and a sea of cars behind me. Taylor was resting safely in her seat and I was a mess. At the time I wasn't firm with my relationship with God, and I was overwhelmed with panic. I did know enough however to give glory to God for his perfect timing. I was grateful that we were "late" and that I was given some sense of warning. Sometimes we are eager to rush and have a plan in mind for ourselves, but it is in His perfect timing and His perfect will that we will be placed in the best possible position. His faithfulness is evidence that no matter what time of day or what situation we are in, He will never leave us. He will guide, protect, and instruct us if we take the time to hear His voice.

My naivety helped me to not fully understand the magnitude of the experience of motherhood. I was somewhat fearless, having little doubt that somehow, we would succeed.

Often the life-changing decisions we make that lead to our most remarkable experiences can be traced back to a defining moment.

My personal experience is not particularly unusual, until one considered the most pivotal decision that shaped my future was born in a small computer lab at the University of Illinois at Chicago. I was a twenty-year-old single mother sitting in a comfortable office chair vigorously typing a term paper. With little less than two hours before I was to board a train back to the suburbs to retrieve my daughter, I had an epiphany. Somewhere halfway through my writing session, I decided that I wanted to be an academic. It was not the self-induced coffee frenzy or the pressure that I felt to complete the word count, but it was the high of accomplishing a goal. I had achieved the level of success necessary in my days of studying quantitative and qualitative research to now complete my essay. However, after this paper was turned in, I knew I was changed forever. It was at that moment that I knew I wanted to conduct research, solve problems, and employ ideas that changed the beliefs of others. Back in those days, my ritual began at 6:00 am. I would wake up in my small apartment and get myself and my special-needs daughter dressed before I called a taxi to transport us to the babysitter. The taxi would drop us off at the sitter just before sunrise. After placing my daughter's carrier in the vestibule of the caregiver's home, I positioned my hands in my pockets and tightened my backpack for the five-block walk to the bus stop. As I waited at the corner for the bus, the concepts for my paper that I would write later that day flowed through my mind, and my enthusiasm for the day's challenges increased.

The University of Illinois at Chicago Campus was in downtown Chicago. My high school was also located near downtown, on Chicago's West Side. It always felt like I was embarking on a daily adventure when

I boarded the blue line train and exited at Racine. I also had a student worker position for the following year. But the first two semesters of my junior year, I concentrated on my classes. Few people knew that I had a daughter and I attempted to fit in as much as possible. I joined the UIC senate and eventually lived on campus the second year. I was thrilled that though my situation was different from a lot of students, I was able to lead a somewhat normal life. I studied when class was over so when I picked Taylor up from the babysitter, I was not preoccupied with homework. That first year went by quickly. I could not completely understand what was happening with Taylor's development. I followed the instructions from therapists and learned exactly what I needed to be an advocate for Taylor.

CHAPTER 2

GOOD FAMILY

I always misunderstood the phrase *good family*. Most people use the phrase when discussing someone's choice in dating. The term "good family" serves as a part of a rubric to follow. My mother would often say, "Make sure he comes from a good family." I thought she meant when dating someone new, I should make sure he came from a family that was financially stable. As an adult I now understand my mother meant something totally different. She meant when a person comes from a good family, then they have a built-in schema for what a positive family interaction looks like.

Every family has their own set of issues and lacks stability in some areas, whether it is mental or emotional. However, there are two common attributes that are present in what I notice in the good families that I interact with, including my own. First, in most good families, there are important traditions that are specific to that one family. Those traditions make up the basic structure of the family and provide them with most of the memories that will serve as a road map for their ongoing relationships. Second, there is good old-fashioned love. Though the dynamics within each family structure varies, those are two key elements that help to make a good family. There are difficult circumstances that occur in all families since no family is free from their fair share of drama and pain. However, a good family knows how to combat those issues with love while continuing to practice those traditions that are unique to their family.

I learned a valuable lesson about self care when I had to spend the holiday alone. I don't remember how it happened. Perhaps I had not created any special plans or came together with friends in time to plan, but we were alone. It was a low point for me. What I wanted more than anything was help. I desperately needed to practice self-care, and it was not the ideal time financially for me to take a trip. It was our first year in our upscale apartment.

People should not be alone. It's scriptural, and when I think of the scriptures, I immediately make them unisex in order to not be offended. I don't think this means that men and women should never be single, but I think it is a truth related to the importance of community.

This means that having a pet, even a fish or a hamster, allows you to care about something else other than yourself. It is important to connect with people daily in order not to become hopeless. My neighbors prevented me from being alone. They were my air and gave me life every time they knocked on the door. One neighbor came by after work and gave me the awesome highlights of her day. I would anticipate her arrival almost daily, and the days she didn't come by it was fine, because every day at 5:15 pm, I trained myself to be ready for her arrival. No matter how stressed I was or what occurred during the day, I made sure my home was clean and ready for company. There is something about the anticipation of friends coming by that drives you to clean and prepare, though she rarely sat down and stayed for more than twenty minutes.

Sometimes, particularly in the winter, those twenty minutes were the only time that people visited us. I had been single for months, and sometimes, that was the only visit I would receive. Though she never knew it, or maybe she did and kept the ritual as a way of caring for me, she created a space for me to breathe. It made me feel normal and was a simple precursor to my long nights. Thankfully during that season, Taylor slept most of the night, but sometimes she would have night terrors or pains and would wake up punching me. It was most likely the gluten attacking her system. To manage my anxiety, I played sermons all night on my broken-down computer and tried dutifully to sleep soundly. When I opened my eyes and realized the sun was up, I was grateful—hopeful for another day despite its challenges and excited to get a visit from my neighbor.

Regarding self care, since then I've learned to listen to my great aunt's advice. Her last words were for me to take care of myself. I remember the last conversation with my aunt very well. She was sick for several weeks, and my mother was by her bedside. She requested to speak with me before going into surgery. We both knew that she may not make it out of surgery, but I girded myself up and stayed strong. As my mother handed her the phone, I listened intently, wanting to respond to whatever she said with care. "Hi Eraina, I love you, you take of yourself, you hear me?" I responded dutifully and as quickly as possible. "Yes, auntie, I will." Those words have stuck with me ever since.

That was some years ago. She never made it out of surgery, and I never heard her voice again. If I close my eyes, I can still imagine what it sounds like. Soft and mellow. One of the most beautiful and deliberate voices I've ever heard. I hope that I have made her proud in how I have taken care of myself. I have yet to master the art of self-care but being a mom of four girls and two bonus boys, an entrepreneur, and a wife, it takes practice. Below are three action steps that I practice in order to take care of myself.

Plan: Sometimes creating a plan seems like a daunting task, especially when you have variables, people, and multiple schedules. But more than planning, I try to stick to the plan. Marking my mental and physical calendar for important dates is crucial. Some dates, events, and appointments are negotiable. Most are not. Though I remain somewhat flexible, even when it is uncomfortable, I keep my commitments. Doing so allows me to trust myself and maintain the trust of others. This is a great way that I take care of myself. Nothing is more stressful than having to rebook constantly.

Rest: Though at the end of most days, many of my tasks on my list are not accomplished, I sleep. Without sleep, I am anxious, moody, and not the nicest to be around. Since I am still breastfeeding my one-year old, and I have a special-needs teenager, even when my sleep is interrupted at night, I go back to sleep. It is one of my favorite ways of caring for myself.

Travel: When I lived on the east coast, day trips were my saving grace. Seeing the highway in front of me was therapeutic. It was helpful to gain a perspective that there was more happening around me than just my physical location or personal life. Traveling expands your view of the world and creates the opportunity to reflect on what is important. Even in small spurts and distances, I try to plan a trip or getaway biweekly. It is also great for the family.

Though they seem simple, this regimen of self-care has sustained me through both great and challenging seasons of my life. If I lack discipline in any of the above areas, I feel it first, and then my family feels it. In the words of my aunt, "Take care of yourself."

CHAPTER 3

ORPHAN

My parents left me. They will tell a different story, but at the age of twenty, I felt abandoned. Being left in a city alone is somewhat like being left in a grocery store aisle by yourself. You look around and nobody's there. Without warning, I was left to fend for myself. Like a lost child, I searched throughout the other aisles one row at a time for something familiar. Once I realized that I was on my own, I launched into survival mode. I still hoped to get a glimpse of my parents. Yet I gathered the tools I would need to continue my journey alone. That is what it felt like, but the truth was I was well equipped. I attended private school since the age of five. I did not lack in the educational foundation needed to survive in society. I was prepared. I was in my sophomore year of college at the time. Though it was awkward to not have anywhere close to call home during the holiday breaks, I managed.

Even at the age of nineteen, I was equipped with housing, education, and a small family network. Their absence plagued my psyche most of my twenties. I was well into my thirties when I realized that it was a path that I had to travel to get where I am now. By the time I was fourteen years old, I felt like I was an only child in my household. My parents were great providers, but they trusted me, thus granting me freedom.

Failing to follow rules was not a challenge for me. I learned early on that good behavior granted tangible incentives. Most of the time I had good behavior, and I loved my freedom. When I became settled in my small Christian Brothers College, my parents moved forward to the next phase of their lives. They bought a lot in an exclusive retirement community in Florida, and within six months, they were gone.

I grew up in a small Midwestern town outside of Chicago. It was a safe working-class neighborhood with streetlights, block parties, and a corner store. Our block was distinctive because though it was made up of bungalows, there were several renovated houses that had add-ons, which made our block seem more unique. One house was named for the character from *Friday the 13th* because no one lived there. Once, when someone appeared to have opened the door, we all screamed and ran down the street in a fit of fear. I stumbled and fell, scraping my chin on the dirty pavement. As I held the bottom of it to stop the gushing blood, I worried about my parents. Would they be upset? How would I explain this fall? As a preteen I felt ashamed, as if I should have known better. They were amazing though, only concerned about my well-being and spared any necessary lectures that could have transpired. I still have a slight scar under my chin, unnoticeable but a constant reminder of that fall. Besides my rocky relationship with my stepfather, I have very few complaints about my childhood. Normal childhood occurrences, like my fall, were commonplace, typical. In hindsight, I was grateful for an invisible bubble-like existence. Though deliberate on the part of my parents, my daily routines, overall safety, and happiness looked effortless to outsiders. It wasn't until I graduated high school that things changed.

My stepdad was strict. There was rarely an action in my household growing up that was not associated with a rule and a rubric. I was great at following rules. Even as an adult, I am conditioned to follow rules. It was the rubric that was challenging. His standard was high, and I never seemed to meet the mark. I would later understand that it was his challenging parentless childhood, young adult years, and limited academic pursuits that fueled his personality and parental style. As a child I just thought he was strict and mean.

In our household we had rules, routines, and chores. From the first day he entered our home, he boldly corrected us and guided us. Again, in hindsight, I understand the pedagogy, the pursuit of a family structure that would yield three adult children capable of taking care of themselves. If I am honest, that is when our good life started.

It was a fall evening in 1986 when my stepdad, in his slick leather jacket, and slightly salt-and-pepper goatee, came over for dinner. There were three of us, my older sister Deila, seven years older than me, my middle brother Brian, and me—the baby, empathetic, sensitive, but fiercely stubborn.

I knew my sister was a leader, even though I was only five years old. My older sister was always respected and mature yet feared. She had put in her time and had endured and remembered everything. Even as a child, I knew she was my protector—responsible yet burdened with the weight of being the oldest. Even my stepfather knew his limits with her. It would take me over thirty years to understand the complexities of her personality, but as a child, I respected her.

We followed her lead without question and unknowingly regarded her as the third parent. I did not see her smile much but hoped there was a sense of joy hidden beneath the surface, and just as fiercely as she regarded her responsibilities as the oldest, her excellent academics, and personal behavior, she was protective of her joy, unwilling to share it so freely. Brian however was a pure ball of innocence. Kind by nature, a responsible follower, only a few years older, he was the perfect big brother. For years, he was the only person besides my father that could calm me down. Until the age of twelve, he smiled a lot, and he was everything that represented goodness and love. As we ate dinner and welcomed this man, a stranger into our home, each one of us played our respective role—Deila the protector, rarely smiley and focusing solely on her meal; Brian grinning from ear to ear, naivety at its best; and me enjoying my meal oblivious to what Deila had already picked up on.

This person was special to my mom and things would never be the same. I remember that he sat at the head of the table. I never saw a man sitting at our table, besides my uncle Junebug. He was more like a sibling than an uncle, eating our cereal and pizza and occasionally sleeping on the sofa for a couple nights a month. He never sat at the head of the table. My dad came over to get us for the weekend or had a meal with us in our home. My parents had been divorced since I was a newborn, and I have no memory besides their wedding pictures of their union.

There was never any major disruption on the street, because at the end of our street and one block over was the police station. Across from the police station was the Park District and a miniature water park called Turtle Island. As I think back, we had a great neighborhood, and though it had some underlying issues, it felt like the safest place in the world, which is why I always wondered why my stepfather set such strict regulations. We were never allowed to go off the block. Our bike riding was limited to our side of the street. We also were summoned in the house when the streetlights came on, and there was little that we could do beyond 7 pm. Sometimes we were in bed so early that we could still hear other children outside playing as we lay in our beds, praying that sleep came sooner than later. Sometimes I would lament over certain rules and regulations that I had growing up. But compared to many people that I have met over the years, I had a great childhood.

My mother has class. She was raised by her maternal great aunt, no blood relation, but she gave her everything her blood did not. My great aunt was an entrepreneur and a businesswoman. Though she lived less than ten blocks from my paternal grandparents, they were polar opposite. Their personalities and traditions varied, but the one thing they had in common was us. They loved us. My great aunt Virginia owned a dry cleaning business on 5th Avenue in Maywood. She was brave and deliberate in her choices, an instinct that she passed down to my mother.

My mother's shining moment came when she joined the team of a well-known cosmetic multilevel marketing company. She did really well too and eventually worked her way up to earning a car. We were thrilled. It was a brand-new Pontiac Grand Am. I still remember how fresh it smelled. The new car smell was distinct, and it was the first new car I remember us having besides our conversion van. With this amazing new opportunity came a red jacket that she and her team members would wear. Her caramel skin tone went perfectly with the jacket, and she was proud and outgoing when she wore it. Naturally an introvert with extrovert tendencies, becoming a part of this new team allowed her to interact with people on a weekly basis, and though we never discussed it, I could tell it boosted her confidence. I watched her get dressed for her meetings, admiring how much pride she took in getting dressed. This was different from her job at the phone company; this was something that she seemed to really love doing. She even had a briefcase that was part of her wardrobe. Almost everything she carried the cosmetics in had that distinct logo. It was beautiful. Her black skirt was a part of the uniform and it looked great. My favorite part of her outfit though was her red lipstick. That's when I knew she had changed; she started to wear red lipstick. At our conservative evangelical church, no one wore lipstick, especially red. I knew then that my mother was brave and that she had stepped into a new dimension, a new freedom. The night she went out was my favorite part of the week, not because she was gone, but because she was always so excited to go and seemed to be so motivated after every meeting.

My father is a tall man. Even as a child, his height was always impressive. His most distinct quality was his confidence and his ability to engage people. He loves to talk, but not just for the sake of talking, he loves to engage in conversation that helps people. He is a natural teacher and a giver. I lived for the two weekends out of the month I spent at his house. I would wait anxiously for his Cadillac to pull up on our street. It felt like I was going away on a retreat of sorts, a vacation from the responsibility of strict rules and timelines. There were expectations at my dad's house for sure, but they were unspoken, and there was an ease with the expectations. He was always excited to see me, and he greeted me with a smile. "Hey girly, girl," he would say. I always felt loved when he walked me to his car, and we headed off even further west for the weekend. My father loved to work. At least that is what it always looked like. His jobs didn't require him to wear a uniform, only a suit. His passion and confidence in corporate America helped to shape my professional relationships and seriousness around the culture of work. One of my favorite memories of my dad is one of the conversations that we had at my grandmother's house during my junior year of college. I was working at a law firm as a law clerk. I loved the position. I was having a tough time with one of the bosses and I wanted to quit. Her microaggressions were unbearable, especially since the hourly wage was low, and technically I didn't need the position. My generous financial aid covered my expenses. "Don't quit your job," he warned. "If you quit, you will encounter the same type of person until you learn to deal with them." He was right as he is about so many things. His ability to strategize and think beyond the situation into the nuances of the problem is a gift.

The reality of my circumstances set in during my senior year of college. I felt completely alone in the city of Chicago. When all the other students left for the summer, me and Taylor were alone in our apartment. We packed our belongings despite having nowhere to go. When we moved in nine months earlier, we thought we had finally settled into a permanent housing situation. The bustling of the students and the excitement of moving into a brand-new dorm were almost too much for the both of us. It was almost unheard of at the University of Illinois at Chicago's campus to have a floor designated strictly for single mothers. The housing department was trying something different. When I heard in the spring there would be a floor designated for single mothers, I jumped at the chance to apply. The area surrounding our building was dusty and barren. It smelled of concrete and debris from the ongoing construction. But when we arrived over the threshold of the front door of the new facility, it was breathtaking.

The smell of fresh paint filled your lungs, and the newness of everything was apparent. New windows, doors, furniture, paintings, elevators—everything was new. We would be the first occupants of the dorm. My new two-bedroom apartment had a handicapped accessible shower, though Taylor was not walking. It was almost a foreshadowing of the days to come. One day Taylor's diagnosis of autism would add a notch to her diagnosis of deafness, making it a dual diagnosis. I appreciated the care that we received during that year at the Maxwell street dorms. At the end of the school year, the single mothers on the second floor received disturbing news. The pilot program for single parent housing was being discontinued. Everyone had to move back home with their children. Accept I had no home. Since my parents lived in Florida, there was nowhere for me and Taylor to stay. That was the first time that I felt like an orphan. All the other women from the floor I lived on had somewhere to go; I did not. It was also a defining moment for me. It was clear this was my family. Taylor and I were a family of two, and it would be an entire decade before that would change. At that moment I vowed two things. I vowed that me and Taylor would never be without a place to stay again. When I had my own family one day, I would never leave them without a home.

My paternal grandmother is the strong matriarch of our family. I did not always understand her approach as a grandparent, but I appreciated the level of freedom I was granted, based on her method of hands-off rearing. Some grandmothers must raise their grandchildren and sometimes their great grandchildren. But Elizabeth Davis was not your typical grandmother. During most of my childhood, she lived directly across the street from my Catholic elementary school. But we did not see her every day. We saw her on Sundays and on the days we were sick. The school would call her to come and get us, and she would pick us up, take us to her home, and feed us our choice of lunch. I always chose a turkey sandwich on white bread, with chicken noodle soup. Those sandwiches were so good. They were made with pure love. She would treat me to a soda and some cookies too.

Her demeanor was always warm. She did not raise her voice. The one time we had a disagreement, she did not allow more than two days to go by before we reconciled. She was my best friend. I never would have made it through those challenging days without her. She was always honest and straightforward. She and my grandfather were like one person and were rarely too far from each other. He would sit in the next room reading the paper, and she would be in the living room, snacking. There was always a television on in their house. Though I never really saw them watching it intently, we mostly talked when I was there. Our conversations were always deliberate and strategic. We would have solved some sort of dilemma by the time our conversation finished.

The new dilemma of the day was my housing situation. Before going over to my grandmother's house for a routine visit, I did not know what I should do. I had no idea where I would live. Again, she was not your typical grandmother, because despite the fact that we had a close relationship, she would never offer for us to stay in her home. I knew this because when I was nine months pregnant with Taylor, she did not offer. Instead she called my father and told him to find us an apartment. He did. He found us a place directly around the block from my grandmother. This time I hoped that she could be equally as resourceful. As I entered the threshold of her home, I immediately felt a weight lifted. I joined them at the dining room table, drowning out the sound of the television, and told them my dilemma.

"Why would they have those girls moved there for only a year?" she asked. "It does not make sense."

"I don't know grandma, but they are all going back home, and I have no home to go to." She was unmoved by that statement as she ate the second half of her bologna sandwich, made with that white Wonder Bread that I loved. I was hungry and hoped that we solved this problem soon so I could go and get a sandwich and some soup and perhaps a chocolate chip cookie. My grandpa always had a stash of cookies.

"Well," she said, wiping crumbs from her mouth and swallowing the remainder of her sandwich, "how much money do you have?"

Since I was not working and the semester had just ended, the only money I had was Taylor's supplementary income from the government. Her check was about five hundred dollars. "I have five hundred dollars."

She nodded in agreement though we had not actually agreed on anything. But I knew better than to point that out. I waited for a verbal response, an answer to my problem. Five hundred dollars was not enough to get an apartment. I would need at least a thousand dollars to secure a safe place in a safe neighborhood. "I will match that," she said. "I will give you five hundred dollars so you can get an apartment." It was like she read my mind. She saw the need and met it. Years later I would understand just how pivotal that moment was. She was fostering my independence. It would take me years to get over my parent's move, but in that moment, I felt that everything would be okay—that though I would not be taken in by family, I would always have a place. I was no longer an orphan.

This entire journey began because I was in search of a good life for my daughter. I was on a quest to finally create a life that was good enough for her and me. Using my own childhood as the rubric, I wanted a life that was as comfortable and carefree as the one I had growing up. As a child I always wanted the best of everything. It is not until I became an adult that I realized that everyone does not share that same passion for the best. I chased after what I referred to as a good life, never fully articulating my plan but striving relentlessly for something better.

Despite moving to three different cities, I pressed on determined not to let my momentary suffering be in vain. Why? I had given up too much and suffered through at least one hungry night. I remember it all, and because I have yet to forget, I cannot really rationalize stopping or giving up. How I remember things is an important part of the story. In fact, all my life stories exist in a collage of selected memories that somehow came together to shape my future. Some memories are too painful to remember, so I block them out. Other memories I replay repeatedly until they stay present in the forefront of my mind.

I was elated that it had finally arrived and resolved to move forward. The next phase of operation *good life* was already underway, and I couldn't wait.

CHAPTER 4

CONCRETE

Several months before Taylor was born, I entered a challenging phase of my life.

It was a sunny afternoon when I met a man who impacted the way I saw the world. He took away my sense of innocence and replaced it with an element of fear. As I crossed the street to walk to the bus stop, he flagged me down and told me how beautiful I was. I blushed because ironically at that moment I felt beautiful. I had just left the beauty shop and my shoulder-length straight hair was blowing in the wind. I was a biweekly regular at my beauty shop ever since I needed phone books to sit at the sink for a shampoo. Her beauty shop was dated and felt like a flashback from the 1970s. The space was huge and sat right across from the fish restaurant that served the best fried fish and chips. Next door to her shop was the bank, and a block away were local shops that had been there for decades, including the business that my maternal aunt used to own. I couldn't believe that I was back in my hometown, though my parents had moved away to Florida the previous fall and my dad lived over forty-five minutes away. I was living only ten minutes away from the hospital where I was born. My khaki-colored overalls were comfortable despite my bulging belly.

I was five months pregnant but clearly attractive to a middle-aged man with freckles.

"Hi beautiful," he said, from his car. It wasn't a flashy car, but it was clean and looked new.

I tried not to be distracted and needed to cross the street safely, especially in my condition, but his car was shiny. My beautician didn't say much about my belly. It was obvious that I was pregnant, and though I grew up in a strict Pentecostal Church, she didn't lecture or judge me. I was appreciative, because it was the last thing I needed. What I needed the most she gave me. I needed to feel beautiful and loved.

As I crossed the street, I pretended not to hear the guy. I pretended that he wasn't flirting, and I ignored the feeling I felt that someone was interested in me, giving me more of what I needed when I went to the beauty shop.

"Hi beautiful," he said again. This time I didn't ignore it. I turned around and smiled. He smiled back, and he had a full set of beautiful straight teeth. He quickly seized the opportunity to connect and rushed out of the car to talk to me. As we stood on the corner, one of the main business strips, he told me about how he wanted to get to know me more. I took his number and left feeling like maybe I would have a friend. After calling him, we met up and connected for dinner.

Being alone in a city with little family was challenging. I was grateful to have my grandmother who pretty much lived right around the block. My dad was still about an hour away, and I saw him twice a month. It left me very vulnerable. And it was challenging to be able to form relationships where I could trust people.

During this season of my life, I learned different lessons about the people I could trust enough to let into my home, how vulnerable Taylor and I were based on our situation, and how I needed to maintain a level of focus and positivity in order to get me through. I tried to date, even when I was nine months pregnant. It was clear that I wouldn't have a relationship with Taylor's dad, so I decided that I would still try to date and form positive relationships. This still proved to be challenging, and even though I created a couple of friendships, it was really challenging to develop romantic relationships that were positive.

Domestic violence is incredibly destructive. It can be stressful for the victim and their family. For me, as a single mom living on my own in a city with little family, I was vulnerable to that type of relationship. One thing I learned about my personal experience with domestic violence is how important it is to share with someone close to you what you are going through. It's very important to create a community so that you will be able to reach out during the challenging times. It's also important to have people to reach out to, whether it's a church or a therapy group that could be able to help you to deal with the issues that cause domestic violence.

In my situation, I was vulnerable, and I knew I wanted someone to be there for me and Taylor. The person that I had the issues with really took advantage of the fact that I was alone. Though it was hard, within a few months, I was able to sever ties in the relationship. But because of that, I learned a lot of valuable lessons. I learned that I needed to be around people that I could trust. I learned that never should I jump into a relationship when I'm in a vulnerable place emotionally or psychologically. As a new mom, as a single mom, and as a full-time student, it was hard for me to make the right positive choices.

The other challenge for me was not having the ability to say no, to shield myself from it. Looking back, I was young, and I was hoping that I was able to create the family that I so craved. I wanted a father for Taylor, and I wanted positive images for us. I don't even understand how we made it through that season. But I do know going forward I was really in the driver's seat for the romantic and friendship type of relationship that I would get in. I didn't have any roommates, and I decided to live on my own, just me and Taylor, and always create a safe and positive environment, a good life for us despite our circumstances.

That was my last physically abusive relationship that I was ever in. After that, I was careful about the people I allowed around me and Taylor. I didn't do much outside in regard to dating over the years because of that incident. I wanted to keep her safe, I promised her that I would also keep her around good people.

It's not easy being a single parent, specifically a single parent of a special-needs child. One day I want to teach other women the importance of having good people around your children. Connecting with good people doesn't mean everything will be perfect, but positive, impactful, nontoxic relationships are so important in order to be successful. My life wasn't normal, but it was good, and I wanted to keep it that way.

CHAPTER 5

ESCAPE

I slept on the floor the night before I left.

I needed to leave Chicago. It was obvious I reached my ceiling of opportunity and it was time to go. It was November of my senior year at the University of Chicago when I applied for Teach for America. I was so excited for the opportunity. I knew in order to leave I must apply for an opportunity to move out of the state. Any opportunity that would pay at least 40k per year was ideal. From what I learned, Teach for America offered a free Master's and the opportunity to teach in an underserved area. I knew I must be deliberate in planning the next stage in my life, and during the time leading up to the big move to NYC I only studied, read, and watch things pertaining to New York. I read *The New Yorker* magazine. I also bought *The New York Times* every day from the Starbucks on Lake Street in Oak Park.

The moment I took my first steps towards moving out of Chicago, everything fell into place. After graduating in the fall of 2002 from the University of Illinois at Chicago, I took a position as a receptionist. As I sat in the lobby at my new job, I knew that there had to be something better than this position for a person with a bachelor's degree. Yet it was not until the spring that I actually walked the stage. Until then, I worked as a temp for a financial advising firm. It was a great experience because it was the means to an end and ultimately propelled me to find something else. After working diligently through undergrad, I was at a crossroads and hoped that I could one day complete a graduate degree program. In order to save money and finalize things before the move, I decided to clean out my apartment. The familiar and former was almost too hard to leave, and during the last two weeks of my stay, I began to become fearful.

By then it was too late; the buttons for my new adventure had already been pushed. We were soon on our way. I drove around completing my errands and visiting friends while listening to my sister's CD player. There was a gospel song I played over and over again. It was all I could do to keep from bailing out of my commitment. Thankfully I could not stay in Chicago even if I wanted. We were camping out in my sister's living room and sleeping on her floor. There was nowhere to go but up, literally. The one thousand dollars I had collected would have to last us while I looked for an apartment for the summer. We had nothing to do but step out. Before our new adventure, I attended Wednesday night service at the church where I had gotten born again at one year prior. I sat still soaking up everything my pastor Bill Winston said, writing down scriptures like a dutiful student who was receiving answers to a future open book test. I also listened intently to the scriptures he referenced when he preached. I wrote my notes on yellow-lined paper, the kind you tear from a legal pad. I knew these scriptures would lead me to where I need to go. They were the best cheat sheet for my next test I would need for the new adventure. I had only one Sunday left before we traveled to NYC. I had already purchased our tickets. Sitting in the congregation allowed me to be filled with motivation, faith, and wisdom.

"There is no use in trying," said Alice, *"one can't believe impossible things."*

"I dare say you haven't had much practice," said the Queen. *"When I was your age I did it for half an hour each day."*

ESCAPE

"Why sometimes, I've believed as many as six impossible things before breakfast..."

(Alice and Wonderland by Lewis Carroll)

The most impactful action I took in preparation was watching a movie called *Disappearing Acts*. It starred Sanaa Lathan and Wesley Snipes. I watched it every single day before I moved. Art imitates life. During that first year I lived in New York City, I lived out the storyline of the movie. I lived in a brownstone apartment in Brooklyn just like the main character in the movie. It felt just like the character that Lathan played; I fell for a rough reformed guy with a past. I was also a teacher working for the New York City Board of Education. Even down to the restaurants and venues they frequented and the romantic intensity of their relationship I lived out. It was eerily similar and reminded me of how much what we watch and listen to have a direct influence on our lives.

My decision to move was prompted one afternoon while I drove to my apartment in a suburb outside of Chicago. As I sat in my Chevy Malibu at the light, I felt that I received the confirmation from God that I should move to New York. I went home, ran up one flight of stairs, and grabbed my Bible. I know that many people talk about an experience of opening up the Bible to the exact scripture that they needed and it appears impossible. It happened to me that day. Before then, I had never officially read the book of Hebrews. This was the first Bible that I ever owned, given to me by my grandmother. And so it started. Hebrews 11. I read the entire chapter aloud. It was like I had a direct line to God.

I knew nothing about New York City initially. I also had no contacts in New York. Thankfully God ordered my steps, because each time I went to NYC before I moved, I met people who would be instrumental once I was there. Things moved quite quickly. From the time I read that scripture in my apartment to the time I landed in NYC late one June night, things moved so fast. When I moved to New York, I did not even own a cell phone. I asked my mother for help. She invested in all my dreams. She knew that somehow things would work out. She booked me a seven-night stay at The New Yorker hotel. It was not a fleabag motel, but on hotels.com, it was the most affordable at $109 per night. From there I had no idea where I was going. I had no one to live with, which meant that in six days and seven nights, I must find an apartment to sub-let—and childcare. The one thing that I did have secured was a job, but it started Monday and I had no one to watch Taylor.

Though she was hearing impaired, her autistic tendencies had not fully set in. She slept ok, and still drank out of a bottle. Since she was a late walker, she was unable to walk for long periods of time, which is why until she was seven, she rode in a stroller. Before I left Chicago, I packed everything that I could into an oversized suitcase. As I neared the hotel room door, I remember how dark it was and how it was in desperate need of renovation. It had a very stale odor and I was afraid of what the room would look like. Our room was in the corner on the seventeenth floor. The security guard looked at me as if I were a runaway. If people mistake Taylor for my little sister now, they must really have thought we were children then. I was twenty three years old and away from home for the first time in my life. As I stuck the key card in, I closed my eyes and waited for the surprise. It wasn't as bad as I thought it would be. It was very small but clean.

The blankets and drapes were crimson and appeared to be identical to the ones hanging in an older person's guest room. It was one of those rooms that felt like a museum display, except it was 2003 and not 1979. I felt like I was stuck in time, somewhere between 1975 and 1980. The furniture looked like it was kept in good shape but from the wrong year. I set my bag down and checked the bathroom. It was tiny and did not include a shower. There was only a small basin and a toilet. I placed Taylor down on the bed and sat on the side of the bed. At that moment the fear did not set in yet. I was still operating from the adrenaline rush because of our plane ride. The taxi ride was also a mini adventure. The driver quizzed me about why I would move to New York. While I should have confessed my unfortunate naivety, instead I told him about how I moved to New York to teach and create a better life for me and my daughter. The look on his face as we exited the taxi was like a concerned parent—fearful yet resigned to let me explore. I checked for my wallet and was somewhat disappointed to know I already started to spend one of the eleven hundred that I had in it. I could not help but hope we would have enough for all the things that we would need for our trip.

I did not have a laptop or a cell phone. The more I sat, the more tired I became. I called my mother from the pay phone in the lobby. She did not sound worried, and I realized now that she was probably just as in shock as I was and did not want to admit it. Finally, fatigue set in and I was in a bed for the first time in a long time. Though I was in an unfamiliar place, it felt very good to finally lie down and sleep on a bed. I checked and double-checked the locks on the hotel doors. From my hotel window, I could see the decks of million-dollar luxury apartments. But our hotel room was far from luxurious. Though I had no friends or family in NY, I had managed to make several contacts when I traveled back and forth for testing.

Though I never left the United States, somehow New York City felt foreign to me. It reminded me of a lesson taught by one of my favorite professors at Yale Divinity. In our Old Testament class, she discussed how two biblical characters dealt with a sense of foreignness. I am in no way comparing my plight to theirs, as we all know the women in the Bible had a lot more to bear than the women in today's era. However, I feel that the three cities I traveled to during the season of raising Taylor left me with a sense of foreignness in various ways. I have mastered the idea of leaving behind something old for something new. I also learn to embrace the seasonal things of life rather than selfishness never wanting things to end. But just as the Bible states in the book of Hebrew chapter 11: If one seeks a homeland, surely you will have the opportunity to return there. But for now, I seek a heavenly home whose builder and make is God.

Looking back on the experiences I had over the years, I must have relied on my faith. There were times when people would ask me why or how I was doing what I was doing, especially during that first year. It was extremely difficult to navigate many aspects of our lives, but I knew I had to do it and for whatever reason, I propelled or even pushed to continue. I think that the most traumatizing aspects of our journey involved the moments where things seemed hopeless and there seemed to be no other way. Each time, God stepped in and there was everything that we needed. For God supplied my needs according to his riches and glory through Christ Jesus. One of my favorite memories of how God supplied our needs was when we lived in the studio sublet that summer.

It was interesting how I even ended up in the sublet. It started back in the spring when I came to NYC for a teaching hiring event. I was standing near the elevator when I met a young eccentric girl who was also in the program. We exchanged numbers and when I arrived in New York, I connected with her. While staying at the New Yorker hotel, two days after arriving in New York City, Taylor and I had managed to run into a major issue. We had no Internet. I had no way of looking up for apartments or sublets, and technically I had two days to find a place to stay. By now I purchased a cheap phone so I needed to go down to the lobby and make phone calls. I looked in my bag, found the number, and called her. Luckily, she answered and was excited to help us.

"Come on over," she said. "I am happy to help you look for an apartment."

We looked over Craigslist under sublet in New York and prayed there were available apartments for sublet. I found one that was in Brooklyn and I called the person.

"Come on over," he said. "I am happy to show you the place."

I found out later, he was subletting this place for a friend who had not yet moved into the building.

"How much you need?" I asked.

"$700," he said.

It was perfect for my budget. I was grateful because it would allow me a few dollars leftover to pay for childcare on Monday. I was grateful for the childcare setup I found in Brooklyn. It was a bit further across town. But little did I know that as I was walking down Malcolm X, dripping with sweat on that hot summer Friday, I was walking in my future neighborhood. I would one day live right off the subway I walked past. God was showing me where I would live one day—Bedford-Stuyvesant. Bedford-Stuyvesant was one of the best neighborhoods I have ever lived in. When I try to explain it to others, I almost stutter because I lack the words to explain the profound impact it had on my life. I called the childcare places I printed out. When I called this facility, they said they were located on Brooklyn. A young man answered the phone and told me how to get there.

"When you walk out of your hotel," he said, "turn right. Cross the street and use the elevator to go down to the A train on the subway. Take the A train toward Brooklyn and continue downtown."

"Where do I get off?" I inquired, as if I would be familiar with the stop anyway.

The first night in our new sublet was scary. It was the first time I felt like I was truly alone. New York is interesting. It is one of the most populated places on the planet, but somehow that night, I felt alone. I was grateful for the double padlock on our door. Two locks made me feel safe. When I asked the super how we should dispose of our trash, he directed me to a trash shoot in the hallway. No matter how often they cleaned the space in the hallway where the garbage shoot was, it always had the smell of bleach, trash, and urine. The elevator was the same, and the worn gate that we needed to use to close it was even scarier. Every time I came in my new place and locked both doors, I felt safe.

It was a wonder that I did not feel hungry that first night. Spiritually I knew it must have been God that took away my hunger because I only had enough Popeyes' chicken for Taylor. Because we had no furniture, we sat on the floor to eat. I could tell she was hungry from how she looked at the three wings. We didn't have enough for fries or anything to drink, but I was grateful. When I purchased the chicken, I was hungry, not knowing how I would split the three wings.

I'd had just enough money to pay for the first installment for our sublet apartment. It was very interesting how I even came to rent the sublet. I jumped in a taxi and headed to Brooklyn. Since we had not been in NYC for more than three days, I was still new to the subway system. We paid a lot of money to get there and I was relieved that we arrived there safely. When the cab pulled up, I was not impressed. In fact, the neighborhood looked a bit sketchy and I was a bit worried. I took Taylor out the cab and made sure to grab her umbrella stroller. That poor stroller probably gained more miles that summer than a rent-a-car. I took that stroller everywhere. I was so grateful to have it, but over the years, because we never owned a car since we moved away from Chicago, I would own three different strollers. "Thanks," I said waving off the cab driver. "I think that this is it." I went into the musty foyer of the building somehow hoping that the inside looked better than the outside. I was disappointed. Luckily, I found an elevator. The apartment was on the fifth floor and I was grateful that there was an elevator.

The elevator was one of those old elevators with the iron gates. I was a bit worried that it would not make it up to the fifth floor, but it did. I pushed Taylor in her stroller down the hall to apartment W. I knocked on the door several times and I even rang a makeshift doorbell. No one answered. I was frustrated because no one answered and I went to knock on the door of a stranger in another apartment. "Hello." He answered. He did not know the person I was looking forward, but it solidified how I was in the right building at least. I was very disappointed and made my way back to our hotel.

I called my prayer partner to help me pray for a placement immediately. I was desperate. It was hard to mask my disappointment, and I wept as I replayed the past two days. I was sad and frustrated things were not working out the way I planned. "Did I make a mistake?" I asked. "Why was I here in the first place?"

She continued to reassure me I made the right decision and reminded me how sometimes even when you are on the right path, things will be challenging. I really had to stay prayed up and not think much about the immediate details of the situation. I had to keep going. There was an interesting exchange the next day between me and the maid cleaning my room. I would not understand until later how again this was a preview or a prophecy of things to come. She was a Spanish-speaking woman who was in my room when I arrived back at the hotel on Sunday. She already made up the bed, and since she was almost finished, I felt like it was fine for me to reenter. I do not even remember how the initial conversation started. Maybe because it was Sunday or maybe because she found scriptures somewhere in my room, but she felt the need to tell me about God and church. The only thing I remember hearing that sounded familiar and memorable was Brooklyn Tabernacle. She was trying to tell me to attend Brooklyn Tabernacle. Weeks later I met another Christian friend on the train who was also in my teaching program. We both later ended up attending Brooklyn Tabernacle together.

God. He was leading me where I would go and giving me a preview of where I should be. Thank you I said, "Gracias."

Years later, while in New Haven, CT, the same thing happened again with another young lady. She also led me to a church, and she was not fluent in English either, but she mentioned God and invited me to her church. After that exchange, I received a phone call from the person I was supposed to meet. I had gotten the apartments mixed up, and though I thought I was to meet him at apartment W, I was really set to meet him at apartment U. I was disappointed and deflated. Thankfully he allowed us to rent the sublet. I was able to move from the hotel to the sublet the following day.

Safety was a common theme throughout my journey. I craved it and worked to achieve it by any means necessary. I needed to feel a sense of safety, even at twenty-four years old. Ironically, the neighborhood where I found Taylor's daycare would be the neighborhood that I would one day live in—Bedford-Stuyvesant, Brooklyn, the home of Biggie Smalls and only a five-minute drive from the famous Marcy projects where Jay-Z supposedly grew up. There was an awesome history associated with one of America's all-black neighborhoods. Before I moved away in 2005, there was a hint of gentrification, but historically since the Great Depression, Bedford-Stuyvesant was mostly black. It bordered the

Hasidic Jewish neighborhood of Williamsburg. On the other side were the already gentrified neighborhoods of Clinton Hills and Fort Greene. I was in awe of brownstones, which held so much history. I might as well have been in another country. I was on foreign ground, a stranger and an outsider to the locals, Including a guy I just met named Quan.

This little girl from the suburbs of Chicago was now rolling through Brooklyn in a 1994 burgundy Suburban with LeQuan. By his own account, he was still awake after losing lots of money gambling on Hancock Street. I met him at the bodega across from the West Indian daycare that I dropped Taylor off at. Now I was riding with him because he offered me a ride. He was more suspicious than I was.

"I could have killed you, Ma," he bragged.

"What are you talking about?" I said in disbelief, still unable to mask my southern drawl. Because everything to a New Yorker was country, even if you had an accent from London, they consider you country.

"You just jumped in the car with me when I offered you a ride?" he said, "I am going to have to teach you a few things."

On the ride to Brooklyn College, the site of my teacher training, he did just that. In those few minutes as we drove to Flatbush, he gave me an education that I will never forget. I was definitely a country girl. I was too trusting and completely unaware of the bad and terrible things that lurked not only in the neighborhood, Brooklyn, or the world. He began to explain how bad Brooklyn was and when I walked down the street, I should not give eye contact to people.

"Don't be so nice, Ma," he explained. "Nod your head and keep it moving, because one day, when you don't speak to them and they think that you are acting funny, they may hurt you. And stop smiling so much," he said. "I understand you are a happy person, but people can take it the wrong way. Because you are beautiful, they will think that they have a chance. Finally, yo', we'll have to work on the way you speak," he admitted.

"The way I speak? What's wrong with the way that I speak?"

"Your accent is way too thick they'll think you're from Alabama, and they will call you a 'Bama."

Now my feelings were hurt; I didn't understand why he was being so blunt and why I had to change the way I spoke. Though I could never really lose my accent, I must make a conscious effort to mask it in some way.

"Ok, let's practice," he said. "Tell me your name and where you're from."

"My name is Errraaainna and I'm from Chicaaaago," I said, clearly unaware that I was being quizzed.

Living in New York City meant that music was all around you. Music from the car radio was blaring out of the speakers as we sped down Stuyvesant. My gut told me that I would be safe with him, that he would protect me, and that I could trust him. I was not as naïve as he made me out to be, and somehow, I knew that he cared for me. Over the next six months, we would have a passionate and intense relationship.

Quan was an alcoholic. He was also a thug that should have been in retirement. The advice he gave was true and accurate because he had been on those streets a long time. He hated Brooklyn. He also hated his life. I met him the day after everything fell apart. I met him the morning after he lost thousands betting on the streets. I was always amazed at how people could lose so much money in such a short time outside the typical casino gambling.

LeQuan. He would be there for me though. Over the next few days, he would take me over on Broadway under the train tracks so that I could buy a futon. Then he would carry the futon up five flights of stairs to a studio sublet that I had for the summer while I studied at Brooklyn College. That summer was difficult and though it seemed like things were not coming together, that is where God blessed me the most. Until recently I had never known a more desperate place of sacrifice.

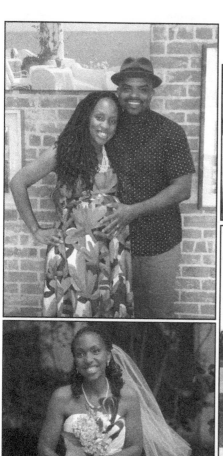

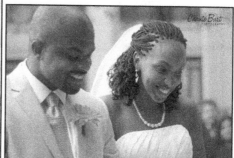

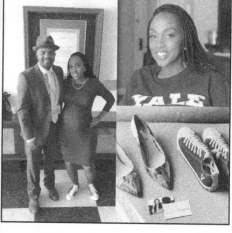

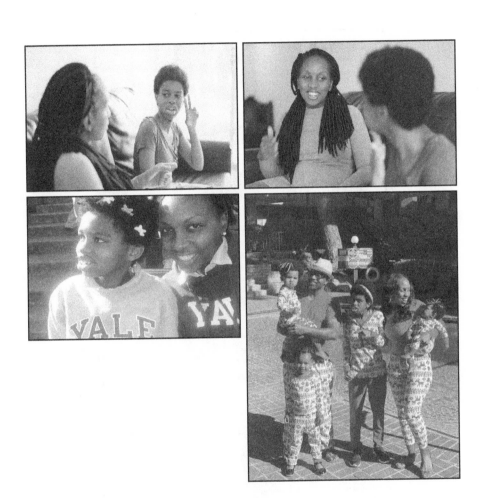

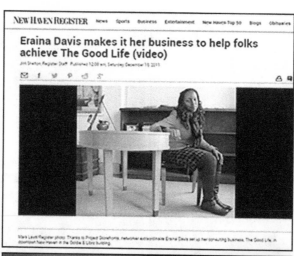

NEW HAVEN REGISTER   News   Sports   Business   Entertainment   New Haven Top 50   Blogs   Obituaries

Eraina Davis makes it her business to help folks achieve The Good Life (video)

Jim Shelton, Register Staff Published 12:00 am, Saturday, December 10, 2011

Mara Lavitt/Register photo: Thanks to Project Storefronts, networker extraordinaire Eraina Davis set up her consulting business, The Good Life, in downtown New Haven in the Goldie & Libro building.

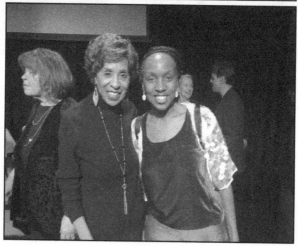

CHAPTER 6

PRIVILEGES

I've always wanted to attend Yale University.

My journey to Yale began back in New York.

In order to appreciate education, you must first despise it.

It all started with Harvard University. My on-again-off-again boyfriend Trevor drove me up 95 North in an effort to regain what we had lost months after our breakup, a breakup so challenging, I contemplated leaving NYC for good.

We met on a Friday evening at Chuck E. Cheese. Me and Taylor took a train and a bus to get to the out-of-the-way location, because there was no resemblance of a children's indoor play space in our neighborhood. Trying to overcompensate for our rocky move and transition to New York, I wanted to make an extra effort to give Taylor a fun experience. I was grateful she was happy, and as she played, I sat at a nearby table, enjoying the quiet.

Trevor, with a suave smile and handsome features, sat nearby and struck up a conversation. I would learn later how it was one of his gifts—the ability to socialize and pull you in, a seemingly innocent charm which would make him a figure in our lives for years to come.

On a brisk cold November day, I fell in love with Cambridge, MA, as I drove from Brooklyn to Massachusetts via 95 North. The fall foliage was magnificent. The orange, brown, and auburn colors appeared to be deliberately drawn onto each leaf. The beauty of fall and it's ever-challenging culture would be what first attracted me to New England. There was something refreshing about the fall season. It begs newness—another opportunity to get it right. It is what I needed, another opportunity to get it right. That first year in NYC was not a complete failure. But between the teaching, Taylor's spiking autism symptoms, and a bad breakup, I was intentional about starting anew. What better place to start than Harvard? Though during my first year of teaching I took classes at Brooklyn College, it was not academically challenging enough. I wanted the opportunity to study elementary education at the graduate level without simultaneously teaching it. I researched programs, and by far, Harvard was the best program in the northeast. The further north I drove, the more beautiful the landscape became. No more concrete sidewalks, only trees, lots of trees, and freshness that welcomed me. The event I attended was a diversity fair for prospective students. My sister attended Brown University. I vividly remembered attending her graduation. It was my first experience at an Ivy League school. There was such a rich history on the east coast. Brown University was nestled in the town of Providence was a perfect beginning to what would turn out as an appreciation for Ivy League institutions for years to come. Since I attended a state school, unlikely for me to receive the opportunity to attend an Ivy League school. Yet I was determined. I felt my grandmothers urging to go for the best; anything was possible. I had gained a new sense of direction and purpose over the summer and now the autumn season begged for something new and fresh. I needed to do my research and listen to the admissions committee regarding my odds for admission. Ironically though I eventually lived in Chestnut Hill and attended Boston College for my Master's, my first experience in Massachusetts was the city of Cambridge, probably the most diverse socioeconomically and ethnically than any other Ivy League town. It was sort of a utopia and offered a false sense of what my life would be like in Chestnut Hill.

Boston was a segregated city, and Cambridge was its apology for segregation, welcoming you with open arms as you drove over the Charles River to a more inclusive and diverse aspect of the commonwealth. Harvard's campus was beautiful. It extended the visual pleasure I received driving on the highway. I was thrilled to attend the diversity open house. Hopefully, this new season would prove to be as rewarding as the drive; scenic and invigorating.

Anything new would also accompany an uneasy and challenging feeling. I experienced it several times over the years. Many experiences offered little introduction but simply a standard by which I was measured despite my current reality. Bringing Taylor with me on these endeavors was a gift but also a challenge. I credit her ability to coexist with me during these outings to her personality. She grew up with me.

Navigating the gorgeous Harvard campus with my special-needs child was humbling. A healthy dose of reality coupled with humility was what I needed during those moments. It was a reminder of my purpose.

My friend accompanied me and kept Taylor while I attended the day-long seminar. The landscape was impressive, and I studied the Harvard logo to see if the visual ignited some special feeling. The detailed mixture of crimson reminded me of the drapes from the hotel we first stayed at when we moved to New York. The gold colors from the logo were eye catching, but I did not swoon over the school. My hope was if nothing else, this experience would teach me to develop a palate for the best while embracing the familiar campus scene. The buildings and architecture were straightforward, nothing spectacular, and almost expected. As I clutched my folder and flipped my straightened hair, which by this time had grown past shoulder length, I surveyed the room, making a conscious effort not to slouch while maintaining a cool posture.

In my survey of the room, I saw several different types of students. Some were already Ivy League students of color, which by this time in history also included Asian-American students, Latino students, students of African descent, my new politically correct term for that time period, and others (students whose ethnic background and nationality were unidentifiable). Everyone wore business casual, which made me grateful for wearing a blouse, skirt, and a fitted blazer.

My beauty supply studs were my latest find, and it was not until I lived in Connecticut that I developed an affinity for pearls. I took a breath and made sure to give eye contact to those that looked my way. I learned the courteous head nod and half smile in my first year in NYC, taught to me by the local thug that gave me many lessons in east coast living. But to show my teeth in a full smile was reserved for people that I knew personally, not for strangers. It would take me years to unlearn my east coast survival behavior. But for now, I followed the protocol, having completely forgotten everything I learned in the Midwest except my manners of course. The thing that I would come to realize about Harvard that I still appreciate to this day is that there is little fluff; the presentation was formatted and deliberate. They never told you more than you needed to know, which is another east coast trait that I adopted quickly.

Sort of like a reporter does, just the facts. Observing the group of prospective students was a lesson in of itself. I learned much of what I needed to know to move forward with my decision. Two very important things were that, first, it was a competitive program for admissions, which means I would need to start studying and retrieving the needed items for admissions, and the second was that though outwardly I looked the part, technically I had a different background than the students represented there; most were east coast educated, by boarding school, day schools, and undergrads. Some of the students there were also legacies. Their parents had attended Harvard, and they were just completing the program, as a requirement, sort of the way people obtain their driver's license. It was what they needed to drive and have access to the road ahead, a preset path of privilege. Neither observation was overwhelming, and as I left the facility, I bounced and walked on my toes with excitement. Two things that I was sure of—I was moving North, away from NYC because the autumn season would be therapy, and also, I would attend an Ivy League university one day, and it all started with Harvard.

I only applied to three schools, and since Harvard was one of them, I decided to apply to two other schools that were in Massachusetts. Before I applied to Boston College, I had never really heard much about it. I did not know that it was a Jesuit College that was started for Catholic Irish immigrants who migrated to the Massachusetts area. When I applied, I originally thought that I wanted to obtain a master's degree that was geared toward teaching high school. The director of admissions who would also qualify to be a part of those good people that I talk about in my corner even then. She advised me to reapply to the MEd for elementary education. She helped redirect my path and that became a vital part of my future at Boston College.

Sitting on that Greyhound from New York City to Boston months later, I could not help but chuckle. I did not fully understand what I was doing next, but I was high with anticipation and uncertainty. I would not discover or verbally admit to my addiction until years later. I was addicted to the newness of moving. There was something refreshing about starting over: new people, new home, and new life. In my mind, I was not running, but was moving forward, most oftentimes led by an opportunity such as school or a new job that propelled me into a new season. It took me away from the familiar. I was still amazed that we were able to fit two years and two apartments into one suitcase. My mind was the carrier of most of our baggage and furniture, and even after years of traveling, the two years that I lived in NYC were unforgettable.

When I first visited Massachusetts, I only visited the city of Cambridge, not Boston. The Boston move, like every major relocation that I would make, was fueled by faith. The woman that I was going to stay with when I arrived in Boston was a stranger. She decided to take us in based on the recommendation of her daughter, a colleague of my former boss. Even then, I realized how establishing good relationships was crucial for success. It was more important that you treat people well than how they treated you. It was a crucial part of my success. As we sat in traffic on the bus ride to Boston, I nodded in and out of sleep, Taylor nestled in the inside seat so I could protect her. The Greyhound was more dangerous to me than a city street at night.

During those early years, I was less aware of the surrounding dangers; but my mother instincts required that I protect her at all cost. Once we were an hour outside of Boston, I became a bit more anxious. The sweet potato pie, and country fried chicken that my neighbor had provided us, was long gone, and I was looking forward to grabbing lunch when we arrived. Ironically, for this relocation we had approximately half of what we had when we arrived in New York City. I had managed to save approximately five hundred dollars for our new trip. Loosely, the plan was still to stay with this woman, whom I would later affectingly call Miss Eleanor, for a couple weeks while we secured housing near Boston College. No Harvard. Though Harvard served as the bait over six months ago when we first visited Massachusetts, I settled on Boston College for a couple reasons, one being that the admissions counselor and I developed a great rapport. She believed in me, and I found out later she submitted me for an academic scholarship that paid my tuition.

According to research, most human beings fall into the category of average intelligence. There are a limited number of people despite their race or background that actually fall into the category of gifted. I am average, as are most people, meaning that I needed to study and read and work. There were some classmates that had a gift for certain aspects of the learning process. They were often bored and able to master a task fairly quickly. I made sure that if it was a concept that I needed to master, I started early and set realistic, small goals. It has been difficult for me to accept that though I strive for excellence, it is difficult to attain because of my circumstances. I never wanted to make any excuses as a student or employee, but there were moments in my career either academic or professional when I just could not reach above the basic requirement. It was just enough. Just good and not great, which is perhaps the reason why I chose that term. Good. Not perfect, not great but good. If one were to give a letter grade, it would be an equivalent to a B+. For some a B+ is exceptional; however, for me it was average. It took years for me to admit that in order to get the A and establish greatness, I had to have a certain number of factors in place: assistance, more time, and more commitment.

As the parent of a child with special needs, it is often impossible to have all of those things at once.

Unfortunately, I did not always have the most in-depth experiences academically, because I was a single parent. At the undergraduate level, I learned to skim well and to pick out the most important information. I also set a goal each night that I would do a realistic amount of academic work within a small window of time.

Most nights I put Taylor to bed at 9:00 pm. I also went to sleep and slept until 3:00 am. I did my work between 3:00 am and 6:00 am. I slept for two hours, woke up, and got Taylor dressed for school and on the school bus. I ate breakfast, and after getting very little sleep, at times, I was propelled mostly by a limited motivation and an even lesser amount of energy. I tried to place the two together to focus so that I could retain the information and summarize sufficiently enough for a positive outcome. My passion for teaching and learning went hand and hand. I loved Boston College. It was just the right size, and in many ways, I enjoyed the graduate experience there more that my own experience as an undergraduate.

When I moved to Boston, I placed Taylor in the Boston public school for the deaf. The school was called Horace Mann School and it was combined with another Boston public school where I would later complete my student teaching. I learned and taught my first lesson at Horace Mann School for the Deaf. Just like with any place I moved; I did my homework. I called the school and chatted with the admissions and special education team.

I explained to them Taylor's diagnosis and they seemed as if they would be able to accommodate her. I arrived in Boston with Taylor's Individualized Education Plan, or her IEP, and I was ready to enroll her in school. On the first day of school, I rolled her up the ramp in her red stroller and went straight to the front office. Though the principal and the special education director knew that Taylor was arriving, they had never formally met her and hence began the worst year of her academic career. When we walked into the office, I inquired about where Taylor's classroom was. I wanted to meet the teacher and get a feel for what their educational philosophy was at the school. I was impressed by our experiences at her school for the deaf in Brooklyn, and I hoped that we would have the same positive experience in Boston. Boston College was about four miles away on what was known in Boston as the "T" train, and I hoped that we could fall into a seamless routine.

"Good morning Ms. Davis; this must be Taylor," said Mr. Ford. "I am Jerry Ford, the principal of Horace Mann."

"Nice to meet you," I said.

We sat down at the front table in office, and I listened for several minutes while he explained why Taylor could not start school yet. I nodded and maintained eye contact as he gave excuses as to why she would not be able to start school. I still did not understand. Finally I interrupted, explaining that because this was a public school, Taylor had the right to be there. Taylor had all the proper paperwork and legally she could not be turned away.

The process had already begun and there was no way that we could or should be turned away. I worked hard not to smile as they excused themselves to decide about admitting Taylor. Part one of the lessons made the first day doable. Preparation is key; when you are prepared and things are in place in advance, good things happen. Though I succeeded in getting her access to the only school that could meet the needs of her dual diagnosis, what I was unaware of was that the teacher was ill prepared for an additional student and her assignment had been changed at the last minute. The school had limited knowledge on how to handle children with autism despite having at least a handful of students on the spectrum.

Many of whom had transferred in the previous year, which is why he attempted to turn us away.

Taylor's first year was a challenge and thankfully she had a teacher's assistant that paid special attention to her. While I excelled academically and socially at Boston College, Taylor struggled to adjust, and I checked in daily with teachers and administrators. The school year was such a challenge that I cried daily worried that Taylor was not receiving an adequate educational experience. After much prayer and advocating, Taylor's second year was great. She excelled academically and socially.

Aside from the beautiful foliage and fresh air at Chestnut Hill, there were other challenges associated with Boston. Demographically, it was much different than New York City. It was naturally segregated, divided deliberately by race, class, and culture. For that reason, it was sometimes a more challenging place to live than New York. Because of those realities, there was an unspoken reality around issues of race in Boston. During a train ride from the city back to our Chestnut Hill apartment, we experienced those differences firsthand. During that season, Taylor's meltdowns related to her autism were much more pronounced. They were louder and more disruptive, and I was new at learning how to conquer them.

The permeating issues around race were related to the forced busing issue during the 1970s. I felt the unspoken issues involving race in Massachusetts. Though I lived there for several years, I was unable to express it fully. However, navigating the unspoken resentment was challenging. In certain instances, it made our time there somewhat uncomfortable. I sunk myself into the Boston College life; I was an eagle now and for Taylor and me, we did what we had done in every new situation.

We joined an affirming community. We continued our road for a good life. Being the parent of a special-needs child is an enormous challenge. There are layers of challenges that faced us daily, and if I was not careful, I would succumb to a life that was not worth living. Ever since Taylor was born, things were a challenge. While I sat in a stranger's home in Jamaica Plains, I reminded myself of how far we had come. The neighborhood was diverse, made up of transplants and liberals and everything in between. The property value was high which made for expensive rent, but the mood was calming and less pretentious than I expected. We were seven blocks from the Mattapan border, and though this would not be our permanent neighborhood, for Taylor and I, it was a good introduction to

Boston. In fact, I had never been to Boston proper; I was introduced to Boston by way of Cambridge on that crisp fall morning when I visited Harvard. Though Cambridge, MA, was different than Boston, JP was not so much different than Cambridge. While still living in Brooklyn, I realized that it was time for me to complete my graduate degree. I had taken a year off because Taylor's diagnosis of autism was given and now it was time for me to go back to school. This time I would go full time in order to complete the task and to get the most out of my experience.

There was little time for one lesson that I have learned over the years involving trust. People are more likely to trust you when you show them that you can be trusted. Navigating the education system involved trust. When you trust people and they fail you, the most valuable lesson that we learn is to trust again. I think that it is so important to dream and imagine those things that we want for ourselves that at times may seem out of reach. It is true that you will only go as far as you think; thus, imagining something big and extraordinary is important, because even if you happen to fall short of the ideal goal, you reached more than you would if you kept a low standard. Having high standards and unrealistic expectations are not healthy. It is good to set both long- and short-term goals, but in moderation you can achieve more than you would have ever dreamed.

After graduating from Boston College in 2007, I had an interesting experience.

I did not plan on staying in Boston and plans of moving to the west coast were foiled. I found myself living in Boston for another year and I was devastated. Fortunately, a friend recommended that I teach at a local preschool that was close to my home. Taylor was settled at Horace Mann School for the Deaf, and we were comfortable in our apartment, located conveniently two miles away from Boston College. Our church was also nearby, which enabled us to still have a sense of community. It was pointless to move; therefore, we stayed in the area and it made sense for me to find a job nearby. I took a position at the local preschool though I was overqualified.

I washed tables, read stories, and packed the backpacks of the

Brookline children, but it was not professionally challenging. It was during that time period that I decided to contact Yale again. However, it was convenient for Taylor and she was happy that I was able to pick her up from school and drop her off every day. It was a good setup, not to mention the fact that I was able to have a clear mind to concentrate on the next thing. It was perfect. While teaching at the preschool, I never let go of my passion for education and my dream of becoming an academic.

I still frequented the university websites and I also looked at my Yale folder often. It was literally a Yale folder, but a folder comprised of things that I had done that summer. It was a memorable summer in New Haven. Though it was one of the most difficult seasons because I did not receive much help, it was rewarding because I followed my passion and my dream of attending my favorite Ivy League school. I also kept a record of the correspondence I had with various Yale professors and ideas about programs that I may want to apply to.

Though I recently graduated from Boston College, I was still looking to obtain a doctorate in order to teach at the college level. The master's in education was more of a practical degree that I could use to teach with, but not an academic degree. I learned this when I went to Yale to visit. My best friend Laura, my only reminder of my Chicago upbringing, watched Taylor while I boarded the train to New Haven; I had met her nearly a decade earlier while volunteering for Amnesty International. She was in law school and lived north of Boston. Taylor and I would spend weekends with her and I was grateful that we reconnected via MySpace that previous year. Our drives north via 95 North were comforting and therapeutic. We would pack up her Subaru with snacks and her dog, Kila, and head north, chasing foliage and adventure. Our race and ethnic differences were never an issue, and our balance of political perspectives gave us a perfect mesh and has contributed to opportunities to learn more about each other over the years.

There is no solid answer to the question of why people suffer. I cannot pretend to understand the motive or the pretense behind suffering. Even after studying theology, I have no inkling as to why people must

55

suffer. I can only tell my account of suffering in a hope to dispel the myth that it only comes in one shape or form. My most memorable experience with suffering was in a one-bedroom sublet in the summer of 2006. This was two years before I would start a graduate program in religion at Yale and while I was finishing up a graduate program in education at Boston College. I enrolled in the course "Civil Rights History and Protest" for the summer of 2006, and I was determined to make this educational experience worthwhile.

That summer was one of the thorniest of my life, and there are days when I try to compare it to other challenging seasons when I realize that it was in a class by itself. There was a moment during that summer when physical pain met pure exhaustion headfirst. The past seven years had been an uphill battle for me as I parented her. As a single parent, I had the task of completing double the work with half the manpower. During that summer, Taylor slept only three hours a night. I was attempting to get some sleep on the modest air mattress that served as our only piece of tangible furniture when Taylor fell backward and our heads collided. It created the most excruciating pain. Taylor seemed unmoved by the incident because lack of empathy and sensory issues are two common traits of children with autism.

For me, the pain was overwhelming and all I could do was cry. That was the bottom for me. I had nothing left. This was a culminating event to the other difficult experiences that plagued us that summer. I did not own a laptop at the time, which meant every other night, I walked ten blocks to the computer lab while pushing Taylor in her red Maclaren stroller. My babysitter was mediocre at best, and I felt though Taylor was safe while I attended class, she was bored and there was a definite language barrier. As I laid there in pain, tears flowing, I wondered what I was doing there, at Yale, in New Haven with no family and friends. At that moment I could not answer that question because I was suffering deeply. At this point the suffering was not just emotional, but physical, and I thought I would die right there on that air mattress and no one would know that I was there. In fact, for many days and nights over the past seven years, all

I had been able to do was cry and ask the simple question, "Why must I suffer so much?"

If I ask my Christian friends, they would say it is because of the "fall." Because Adam ate that damn piece of fruit, an apple or a pear or whatever it was. Because of him I must suffer. That answer is not good enough for me. One day I would be able to think clearly and realize that all of the suffering, the sleepless nights, the physical pain, and the stress, balanced by various instances of happiness and windfalls of blessings, were all a part of the plan. Despite the pain and agony that I felt in that moment, I pressed forward. I arose from the air mattress slowly, dried my tears, and kept going. I would complete this cycle for so many days after: first pain, then tears, then moving on. No matter how badly I felt now, I had no one to help and I knew that I must keep going. I was determined to not make Taylor's disabilities an excuse to live below what I deemed a good life. I was determined to do my best even when I knew it was not good enough, knowing intuitively that if I had gotten more rest, I could have done just as well and accomplished even more than the average person. Over the years, I have done the best I could to mask the internal pain with an external smile in a hope that no one could see that I was suffering so much on the inside.

Waiting for a season of suffering to end is similar to waiting on a thunderstorm to pass. It reminds me of a night during that same summer of 2006. The night was dark and stormy. Taylor and I had finally arrived at the computer lab on Elm Street, past the New Haven Green and the Yale music building,(almost over the river and through the woods. As she was asleep in her stroller, I typed my assignment that was due the next day. After completing my assignment in the lab, we walked outside and into the storm. We headed to the student bus stop. I frantically pressed the button on the call box and waited. I listened to the recording on the other end, but through the static, I could barely make out what they were saying.

The thunder and lightning did little to help make this call clearer, and the rain pounding on my umbrella seemed to reiterate the urgency of this call. I was worried that the person on the other end did not hear me, so I called again and belted out the same plea, "I am at the twenty-four computer lab at the engineering building, could someone please come get us, and does anyone hear me? We're going to York Street." I knew that I must have faith and patience, trusting someone heard our desperate pleas and was sending a van over to rescue us from the storm. My patience dwindled with every drop of rain and clash of thunder that passed. I prayed they heard us and that the bus would come. God gave me the faith, patience, and endurance to wait out the storm until help did indeed arrive. Just like the wave of suffering that life brings, eventually we were rescued, and the storm passed.

I love to travel. Movement has always served as an adrenaline rush for me. I prefer the train because it is always moving in one direction. Though it pauses for a bit along the way, there is a set destination, and psychologically movement allows me to have a sense of direction. Perhaps it is the freedom and the anticipation of the next thing. Staying in one place allows for a sense of monotony. Traveling also allows for new experiences and new people. It helps me to breathe.

I love the train because I can move at a fast pace without doing any of the work. Looking at the beautiful scenery outside the window is refreshing. I have traveled often via train between the three different cities over the past seven years—New York, Boston, and New Haven, each city bringing a new set of challenges and experiences. I would not change a thing about the places I have been or the people I have met along that way. I once took the train when Taylor was a baby from New York to Chicago and back again. On the way back to New York, the train was stopped at around ten o'clock that night. When we woke up the next morning, we were in that same spot. I was not upset because our train was delayed or because I was worried about traveling with my young child, but because we were stopped in the same spot without movement for such a long time. The stagnation was almost paralyzing. I am con-stantly seeking ways to move. However, sometimes a period of standing still is important for growth. I was grateful that we eventually made it to our destination at the appointed time with everything intact. I must learn to appreciate those times. Standing still waiting for movement is an inevitable part of life.

I travel not to go anywhere, but to go. I travel for travel's sake. The great affair is to move.

(Robert Louis Stevenson)

The train always provided a sense of solace. The east coast is filled with many opportunities to commute via train. The day trip to Yale was supposed to be an opportunity to interview for a doctoral program. After presenting at the Yale Bouchet conference and attending Yale summer school, I knew it was where I wanted to be for more academic training.

I went back to Yale in the spring of 2007 before graduating from Boston College to present at the Bouchet conference. My topic discussed the need for diversity in the academy. Though it was only a student-ran conference, it was a great opportunity for me to present the preliminary research I conducted on diversity in academia. I invited a mentor from New York, and Taylor and I stayed at the Holiday Inn on Whalley Avenue. I even saw my barber from the previous summer, and he gave me a fresh lining for my presentation. My friends took the train in from New York to see me present. It was a great experience. I was so happy, and it felt natural for me to present in front of a classroom of peers and fellow students. We had dinner at The Graduate Club on Elm Street. It was a perfect day. As I looked through the folder at the handouts, I was reminded of those dreams I had of attending Yale for graduate school. I telephoned the administrative assistant from the conference and she gave me a simple instruction that would change my life. Whatever program you would like to attend, simply email the professors. It was a life-changing statement because she supported my passion and gave me positive basic advice that helped me to decide on the next good memory.

Historians have often been intrigued by the many facets of memory and how memories are categorized and compiled. For me, my memories of the past seven years are often difficult to retell. There are specific ones that are easy to remember, and if I close my eyes and think back, I almost feel like I am in that place. Others are too painful to remember; I keep them in a secret place and I wonder if I will ever be able to tell them. Living on your own at such a young age is difficult and taxing. Most people have family and friends to support them in their endeavors, to give them moral support and encourage them. I had to make relationships from scratch, sometimes taking chances on people hoping that they did not hurt me in the process. When you are a transplant, you have no history in a particular location. No roots. You must research, network, and start over.

CHAPTER 7

GOOD LOVE

There is something amazing about love. It holds you close and makes you feel safe. Never failing. Never wanting anything. Always steady. There is something even better about being cared for. Adored. Loved. Real love and good love can sustain you and keep you safe from harm. Good love is authentic. Powerful. Good love + more good love = a good life.

> Love is the immortal flow of energy that nourishes, extends and preserves. Its eternal goal is life.
>
> *(Smiley Blanton)*

After dating off and on for twelve years, I finally found love. I embraced it, enjoyed the good, and let it restore everything that I thought I'd lost forever: family.

The first time I met Jason, I remember seeing him on the basketball court. He was running up and down the court and he looked so confident and at peace. I knew he was popular, but I didn't have the desire to necessarily get to know him. I was a cheerleader in high school, and it was important for me to focus on academics. I felt like cheerleading was a job

I was hired for. I loved to cheer on people, give them support, and help create an environment for them to win.

I was moderately popular. There were other students more popular than me, like the head of the cheerleading team and the pom-pom team. But I felt like I had a good middle ground. I only had two friends I was close to at the time, and they happened to not be in the same class as me. They were a year behind me. My high school years were great. At one point my aunt was the dean of students. I was confident I had a good base, and I felt like I was liked by most people.

The hardest thing about my high school years was my commute and from school. My mom brought me to school daily. On her way down-town to her job at the phone company, she dropped me off at school. On my way home, I had to walk two blocks to the bus stop and then take a bus all the way to a train. I had to take the train home and take another bus home. I learned a long time ago, when you want something, you must work hard for it. Sometimes there will be struggles in between and there will be sacrifice, but it will be worth it.

By the time I made it to my senior year, I felt great. I was ready for college. When it was time, we were able to apply online for our colleges. We had to use a new system. AOL and the internet were just starting to boom.

It was 1997, and I felt like this was a year to take my life to the next level. My sister was brilliant, and she had graduated years before me and set a precedent that I didn't feel like I could be able to replicate. She was valedictorian and she also was a first-generation Ivy League student at Brown University.

When they scanned our applications and gave us the option of the schools we would be able to attend or apply to, I knew that I needed to cast my net wide. I applied to five schools and was accepted to several. The school I decided to attend was Lewis University. It was a Christian Brothers School located forty-five minutes south of Chicago. I knew college was going to be different, but I was excited to accept the challenge.

It wasn't until years later that I reconnected with Jason. Though we had gone to school together, I had no reason to talk to him before we reconnected in 2011. Facebook created such a plethora of options to connect with alumni from my high school. I became friends with hundreds of alumni before and after the years that I attended. Jason was no different. I moderately looked at his profile. I couldn't really tell much about him from it. I wrote a blog post about teamwork that resonated with him. I thought he would appreciate it because it created the memory for me of cheering him on in high school. I sent him the blog and he responded in a positive way. He was very humble and excited that I would include our story of me cheering on the basketball team in a blog post.

We moderately conversed via our inbox and that is when a friendship started. He reached out and said one day he'd like to talk more about me and my daughter, Taylor. I was one year out of Yale and living in a doorman building in downtown New Haven. Still a single mom, I dated sporadically but nothing serious. When he decided he wanted to talk to me, I scheduled time. I knew I wanted to be able to give him something tangible. One thing I noticed about him the most was how he would write deep Facebook posts. For his brand, I felt he needed his own blog or his own website.

We talked on the phone and he felt like he could do anything after our conversation. I talked to him about what I thought about him creating a blog, and gave him the password and login for it so he could one day just create his own website. I saw him as a leader and an influencer before the word influencer was a buzzword.

When we got off the phone we both felt good. A month later, in August of 2011, he called me when he was at his family reunion and reached out just to say hello. It was great to hear his voice, and it felt like this could really bloom into something special.

Several weeks later, I hit a really low point emotionally. It felt like one of the worst weekends of my life. It was on the Friday before Labor Day. At the end of August, right before the Labor Day weekend, me and Taylor were in our apartment and I had her home for about a month at that time. I built up the stamina to have her for four weeks and for us to do our daily regimen of her bedtime, eating, restaurants, libraries, and, of course, the Barnes & Noble Book Store. We still had the opportunity to hang out at Yale's campus though I was no longer a student.

Then I received a call on Friday that changed everything. It was low point for me. It was a robocall from the school saying she could not start school on Monday or Tuesday because of the weather. I was distraught. I was devastated. I didn't understand. I knew it was clearly a concern for weather reports, but what it felt like to me was yet one more day I would have to serve as a caregiver with little support. It wasn't until that moment when tears flowed for about ten hours that I knew that I had hit a low point of exhaustion.

I reached out to a friend because I was concerned. I thought I was having a nervous breakdown. I was having panic attacks throughout the day. I couldn't stop. I didn't understand why I was so upset. But it was clear in a lot of ways I was at a point where I needed more help. II prayed to God for help, and for someone who could come to help me raise Taylor. I reached the limit. It had been eleven years, twelve years on my own. I knew this was the time that I needed to be able to have support. I dried my tears and went to sleep. I woke up the next day and we boarded a train to Brooklyn to visit my cousin. I knew that a weekend trip away was exactly what I needed to have a change of scenery and to breathe. I slept on her sofa and rested. She was doing her residency in Brooklyn, and it was great to be able to have family nearby.

During my weekend my weekend away, I received an unexpected call from Jason. It was kind of a short call and he was confident in his tone. Maybe he felt something special, I knew we both were connected. He said, "You know what Eraina? I think I'm going to try to make a trip up to the East Coast." I took it with a grain of salt because a lot of times men will say things and, I don't know, I just wasn't trusting it. I felt like they always have the desire to prove something extra when they come visit. As I listened to him, I felt good about our conversation. When I got off the phone with Jason, I immediately felt better, but I knew I still needed help. Him coming a month later even as a friend didn't really mean anything for my current reality.

Monday arrived and it was time to go back to New Haven. I knew Taylor would start back to school and things would get better immediately. I was set to start working as a Policy Research Analyst for the University of Connecticut, and I was excited. But first, I needed a rest.

When I put Taylor on the school bus, I received a call from Jason again. I answered, excited, thinking that he would have some great updates on what he was working on. But what he said changed my life.

"Hey, Eraina, I actually have some good news."

"What's that, Jay?"

"I was asked by the University to accompany a group of student leaders to New York in October in order to help out for a field trip for students."

We were both equally amazed. It was September 1st of 2011. That day changed both of our lives forever, because we knew we needed to talk, and we knew we were connected and maybe we had a shot, and we held onto it.

From that day forward, we talked on the phone for hours everyday. I was able to go through his life and he was able to go through my life by talking on the phone and figuring out what we did each day. Every morning he woke up at 5:00 am to start his two hour commute to work. He worked hard throughout the day as an administrator at Chicago State University, and I was starting my position virtually as a research analyst at the University of Connecticut.

We also prayed over the phone together. We took our friendship seriously. Day by day we started to develop feelings. We told our stories. We were raw and passionate. We felt this connection and started to bond almost instantly. As the days got closer to our in person visit we became more excited. His birthday was on October 12th, and I even sent him a gift. I was excited for him to come visit me.

Besides having the University of Connecticut Policy Research position, I was offered the opportunity to open up a storefront in downtown

New Haven, literally across the street from my building. He was able to support me. He gave me encouraging words and got excited about the opportunity for me to give other people advice. I knew when I received the opportunity to open a storefront, I needed to call it something special. As I crossed the street with the city of New Haven administrator, she asked me an important question, "What will you call this store?" And I said, "Good Life."

As we developed our friendship, we became more excited that soon we would finally be able to see each other. I gave my cousin a heads-up, letting her know I would need her to watch Taylor because I was going on a date with Jason Ferguson, *Jason Ferguson*. I was so excited. It was important to me to be able to connect to him physically and not just over the phone.

When the weekend finally arrived, I was more than excited. I packed our bags. I did my hair. I was thrilled. I was a little nervous about him meeting Taylor, but I knew I needed to see him, and once I saw him, I would know if this was something I would want to continue. My cousin was great, and it was on a Friday evening when Jason decided to take the train down to Brooklyn to see me. His hotel in Manhattan was filled with students, and he was able to get away in the evening just to come and hang out.

When the doorbell rang, I was so nervous. I went to the door and I opened it up, and there he was. He had on a newsboy hat and the sweater that I bought him from J. Crew. It was black with white stripes on it. It fit perfectly. When I opened the door and I looked at him, I felt a connection because we had been talking for so long for the past thirty to forty-five days and I knew that something special started to build. I decided no matter what, we would be friends. When he opened the door, he hugged me tight, he hugged me as if he never wanted to let me go, and I knew this was it. It was something special. We both smiled as we headed off to our adventure. We left and boarded the train towards Downtown Brooklyn. I wanted to show him some of my favorite parts. I hadn't lived there since 2005, but it was still a very important place to me.

We went to one of my favorite streets, Montague Street. Montague had everything on it. Some of Brooklyn's best restaurants were on Montague Street. It was also blocks away from the promenade where you could see the space where the twin towers once stood. We went to an Italian restaurant I had never been to before. As we sat down to eat our salads, we were both blushing. We were eating salads because we were fasting. We were so set on making sure we did this thing right, we decided to do a spiritual Daniel fast. We ate our salads and smiled and talked. In this Italian restaurant where contemporary music usually played, our favorite rhythm and blues song came one. It was almost like God was giving us a sign that we were on the right track. During our talks, we'd talked about music, we'd talked about love, and we'd talked about our spiritual beliefs, but we also connected over Ray Charles. There was a song called *I Got a Woman*, and it came on. We looked at each other like, "What? In this small mom and pop Italian restaurant and this song would come on?" We were shocked.

We still enjoyed our meal and we savored it, and when we left, we walked down the street holding hands like it was some movie. I showed him all the places me and Taylor had been before, and a lot of things that we connected around. When it was time for him to take me back, we hopped on the train together; he went back to his hotel and I went back to my cousin's house. I knew whatever time I had with him was valuable. We had a date the next day too, and then when the time came for us to end our weekend, we were both sad. But I was confident something more would happen. I promised him when November 1st came, I would buy a ticket to Chicago.

This was a huge deal because little did he know, but I had trauma and hurt and pain around the city of Chicago. Since my parents left in 1998, I hadn't really had a strong relationship with the city. Being there on my own for those couple of years raising Taylor alone was traumatizing. I was on my own, and it was hard, and even though I had the help of my dad and my grandmother, it was still a lonely place for me. When I went back to visit year after year, every time something bad happened or a connection with someone I used to know didn't go well. It was not a happy place for me, and though the year was 2011, I hadn't been in Chicago since 2009. But I was willing to go back to see if this was a place I could at least visit or live in for a short span.

I knew it was far-fetched for Jason to move out to New Haven, so in my mind I decided if I go to Chicago for Thanksgiving and it's a positive experience, I would consider a short stint there. On November 1st I purchased my ticket. I was at peace because I really had the opportunity to go and see and explore what Chicago could be for us. We spent Thanksgiving weekend together. I was able to see his townhouse in the suburbs of Chicago and we had a great time. I visited his church, and I met some of his family. It was a great time for me, but most importantly, he got to meet my father.

They connected immediately and my dad remembered being in the stands and seeing Jason on the court when I was in cheerleading. He would commute in the evenings when I was in high school and come out and sit in the stands just to watch me cheer on the sidelines. It meant so much to me. He knew who Jason was and he was thrilled they had a little bit of the same career path. Though Jason was an administrator at a college, he was also in emergency management.

Moving to Chicago became more emotionally and physically taxing than I first thought. It was the dead of winter in January of 2012. Though for the most part it was a good transition with moving into my apartment, psychologically I had to prepare myself for a completely different fight regarding education. This would prove to be one of the most challenging seasons advocating for the right educational system for Taylor.

Chicago was way behind major cities like Boston and New York when it came to education for typical children, let alone for special needs. Taylor somehow was placed in a school that didn't have any students who were deaf and barely had a special education class to meet Taylor's needs. Before I knew it, I was spending hundreds of dollars per week to take a Zipcar back and forth to school and connect with the teacher, all to no avail. I worked hard to cultivate a relationship, and in the end, I ended up having to connect with the superintendent of Chicago Public Schools and their major systems, because the teacher called a meeting to put Taylor in a program that was more like a mental institution. It was a nightmare. It was heartbreaking, but it also confirmed why I decided to leave Chicago years ago. It was one of the seasons I realized how though you can cultivate a close relationship with the education system and your child's school, inevitably it can all fail in the blink of an eye. It can feel like your hard work was for nothing.

The upside to that season was between January and June, Jason and I dated, and our courtship was amazing. We were able to be in the same city, eat meals together, hang out, do events, and really get to know each other for the day-to-day level and not just over the phone. If anything, it validated how we were on the right track and we would build something great. It was just me, him, and Taylor, our cool meals, and our downtown excursions. I was able to plug into the community in the South Loop area.

By June, we were at a crossroads because I had only gotten a six-month lease on my apartment. I knew soon we would need to decide: do I go back to New Haven, or do I stay? I wasn't staying as just a girlfriend. I would need to be a wife. I set the standard verbally and even psychologically for myself, so I didn't stay in the city for too long, and so I didn't develop a resentment for our relationship, and it didn't feel heavy. It always felt light and easy, and we created this spreadsheet and planned.

We got down on our hands and knees on the floor and sat and wrote out on post-it paper what we wanted over the next three months. It would take years until we realized that this was probably the best method for us. Write a scope and sequence of what our expectations were, put it in front of us so we could plan it, and that's what we did. We planned the next three months out with major events and a checklist with that we needed. We plastered it on the wall of my apartment loft, and we looked at it.

On July 12th of 2012 Jason proposed. We got married on August 17th. He got down on one knee and sang at an amazing spot at the observatory at Northwestern University. It was a beautiful moment, and six weeks later, we were married in a wonderful wedding of 100 people, our closest friends and family. It was in downtown Chicago literally blocks away from where my loft was. It was a wonderful event, and even the days leading up to that, God orchestrated it all. Jason gave me a $5,000 on a debit card and told me to go for it. Even though it was intense and sometimes stressful, having that small time of engagement was probably the best bet for us.

I went back to the same place in Evanston where Jason had proposed to find us an apartment. I drove up to Evanston hoping to find a great place. I parked in front of an apartment building that inevitably had a sign, and I was led to it because that was around the block from the coffee shop that we had gone to right before Jason proposed. I had seen a realty place that I felt like I should go to, so parked in front of this space, and I felt like, "Okay, let me just call this number." Who knew that apartment on the second floor would be where we would live?

We moved in after we got married, and it became one of the best spaces for us to cultivate our newlywed year. Evanston was great. It was a utopia of sorts, a diverse small-town right in a college town at its best. Ironically, those were the towns me and Taylor had thrived in over the years. Our college town in Boston and our college town in New Haven felt like safe spaces, and they felt like they were cultivated just for us. It was a bonus to plug into a university too.

It was a walking town, and Jason eventually landed a position at a consulting firm blocks away. We had our going away party in a mansion down the street from our apartment. Our first year of marriage had all the cool things that occur within your first year: getting to know each other, job changes and planning yet another move. At the beginning of the summer of the following year, we were expecting a baby, and Jason accepted a job offer in Los Angeles, California. This turn of events created a perfect environment for us to build our new life, and in tow with baby five months in utero and Taylor with us, we boarded a one way flight to Los Angeles, excited about our new adventure.

Again, our next year in Los Angeles and the years after would prove to be the same formula: planning, stepping out on faith, creating a job environment that worked for our family, and building. In between those times, we had more babies, more little ones.. We were so grateful for the opportunity to build our small and deliberate family.

Building an abundant family along the way and creating the friendship helped me shape my good love. Building a family and making sacrifices and changes towards my good life has not been easy. Originally, when I walked out of the hospital with Taylor, it was just us. I didn't have to consider anyone else. My hopes were my hopes, my dreams were my dreams, my successes were my successes, and my failures were my failures. Cultivating a good life while in a partnership has been challenging, but it's all what makes up our good life.

I would never regret the decision of partnering with Jason. His good love has helped me grow, has shown me the face of God, and has inevitably allowed me to create legacies of beautiful little ones. We are able to instill those same things that help us cultivate our love over the years. Our life isn't normal, but it's good.

CHAPTER 8

EVER AFTER

After getting married, I became aware of the beauty of partnership and the new dynamics of family. I also discovered new things as a wife and mother of two more children. Raising a child with special needs and building a family was not easy. I discovered that this isn't a normal life, it's a good life.

"Mommy, Taylor fell down." Those words would haunt us for a long time. Our toddler repeated them for months after the incident. As we looked over to figure out what happened, things seem to move in slow motion. Taylor had fallen on the floor while watching television. She was convulsing and having what looked like a seizure. We immediately place her on her back and made sure her airway was clear. We started to pray out loud, and we sent our toddler to her room. We moved to Texas several months before for Jason's job. As people of color, we knew we were not even safe in our own home and needed to create an environment of calm. It felt like a long time, probably eight minutes for the ambulance to arrive. Even though we were in our own home, I took out my ID and my insurance card.

We learned at the hospital Taylor had a grand mal seizure. Though she was diagnosed with deafness at birth, and autism at the age of five, she had never had a seizure. Even though I was afraid, I got dressed and loaded my toddler and infant into the car and headed to the hospital. I was more shocked than anything. The doctors conducted exams. After receiving the results of her CT exam, we learned she did not have a have a mass on her brain or any abnormal growths. The only thing that the CT showed was her cochlear implant, which she had been given years prior. Epilepsy does not run in our family. The only thing we knew was how some children with autism develop onset epilepsy as they enter adulthood. The diagnosis was troubling because Taylor had overcome so much.

This new aspect of our journey was what reminded us of the importance of family. We were building something we hoped would last, and we protected our family and marriage with everything we had.

After Taylor's seizure, we planned an impromptu road trip to Chicago. On our visit to Chicago, we went by Taylor's dad's home and he was able to meet my other two children and see Taylor for the first time in years. She remembered the house and sat on the sofa with excitement. She knew he was her father, and she was elated that we were able to hang out with him. Months earlier Kevin had reached out and expressed a desire to connect with Jason. Kevin felt that Jason was probably cool and a great guy. He was right; without reluctance, Jason reached out and he and Kevin developed a friendship. First Kevin wanted to know how Taylor was doing and was grateful to have check-ins with Jason about her health and academic progress.

Having grown up in a blended family, it all made sense. It was only right that Kevin have access to Taylor, and just because we weren't extremely close didn't mean him and Jason could not have a connection.

There were key steps I needed to do to help me forgive him.

When I gave birth to my daughter Taylor at the age of twenty, I knew that there would be some challenges. She was born with severe hearing loss and displayed global developmental delay almost instantly. Her father's lack of involvement compounded with her special needs created a sense of resentment and anger.

However, after sixteen years I was finally able to forgive my daughter's father for his absence. I followed the following steps to come to a place of peace to forgive.

I forgave myself.

It takes two people to create a child. Though I was nineteen when I became pregnant, I was aware of what would happen if I did not practice safe sex. I was not a victim. As a sophomore in undergrad, I was thankful for my family and friends who supported me while I worked hard to finish school. Owning my choices allowed me to replay the details of our relationship without casting blame. I made plenty of mistakes in my desire to have a father for my daughter. Part of starting the healing process involved owning my choices: the good ones and the bad ones.

I moved on.

Once I realized that my daughter's father would not be involved to the extent that I needed, I moved on, first, emotionally and then second, physically. I moved thousands of miles away and started a new life. I pursued my dreams and passions to the fullest without regret. The decision to move on was not difficult once I faced the reality of what his involvement would be. My success was never contingent upon his involvement. I had freedom. Engaging my freedom meant embracing the limitless choices life brought my way. I dated, traveled, completed school, married, and eventually built a life for myself. My husband is a loving dad and provider for my daughter. Moving on helped tremendously with the forgiveness process.

I saw the good.

I was deliberate about seeing the good. Another step toward forgiveness involved me extracting the good from the situation. A good aspect of the situation besides my awesome daughter was additional family. Her father's family displayed remarkable kindness and acceptance from the very beginning. They always made it clear that they loved Taylor. Their involvement helped balance the rejection I felt at the beginning. The other piece of good I recognized early on was the level of freedom I had to make major decisions regarding my daughter's well-being.

Since she was born deaf and was diagnosed with autism at the age of five, there were many decisions I had to make on my own. Though some would view this as a limitation, I saw it as a good thing. Because of his lack of involvement, along with the consultation of doctors, I had full agency to make decisions regarding her progress. One decision included a surgery which helped restore hearing through the implantation of a cochlear implant. I also had the freedom to move out of state and pursue graduate school. Absence is not always a bad thing. There is freedom in limited involvement.

She lacked nothing.

Despite my daughter's limited understanding of her father's lack of involvement, she was afforded the best of everything I was able to give. Though I often overcompensated in certain instances, especially during holidays and birthdays, I was grateful that she had everything she needed. Thankfully over the last 20 years, we were able to create a village of people who were affirming and loving toward us. She attended schools and programs that met her needs while gaining exposure to new experiences. I even found an amazing skiing program for special-needs children in Maine, and she traveled with me to at least three university campuses during my time in graduate school.

I heard a sermon by Touré Roberts that helped free me from the last bit of hurt. In the sermon, Pastor Roberts describes three kinds of fathers. When he mentioned the father who was never involved but still loves his child, it helped me release the last bit of hurt. Over the last few years, though I had completed the above steps, I felt obligated to hold on to a little anger since she is not able to express it herself. Somehow, I was filled with a peaceful resolve that he loved her, despite his choices.

Love wins.

My spiritual beliefs helped me to understand the power of love. It always wins. Over time, I was able to realize that the same love that I feel daily from God is the same love that would help me to forgive her father. Forgiveness doesn't mean that you become best friends with the person, but it releases the level of hurt and anger that keeps you tied to them emotionally. When you forgive, everyone wins.

My Good Life Now

I couldn't believe where I was.. I was headed to the WACO Theatre, an exclusive theatre in North Hollywood, where I would hear my monologue being read by a famous actress. Per usual, with our growing family, it took a lot to get there. We coordinated two babysitters for our four girls, one of whom was with us. I am thankful our stage nanny accompanied us when we had filming gigs or appearances. Since our daughter Winnie was so young, I loved to keep her close to us, and I'd done the usual in preparing for the day, timing our day deliberately in order not to overlap with too many other events. The morning of the event, I had the opportunity to do what I love: give self-care services to moms of special-needs children.

My Good Life received its 501c3 status three weeks prior, and now we could officially be a giving organization aimed at giving self-care activities for families with special-needs children. As I gazed out the window, breathing and taking it all in, I was overwhelmed with gratitude. If someone had told me one day, I would be able to give what I was so badly in need of two decades ago, I wouldn't have believed them. I knew the entire time my commitment was to serve others. I knew for some reason, me and Taylor were chosen, and through no effort of our own, doors, large doors were opened on our behalf. At some of the most interesting pivots of my life, I received good news and good opportunities. Those chances, sometimes second and third chances, were not given by accident. Without knowing who would read my monologue, I walked into the theater and sat in row F. I'd purchased the entire row because my husband's aunt and uncle, our Hollywood parents, were joining us. Their support and excitement for my success was apparent, and they loved the arts, theater, and performance.

They still worked hard on their solo and collective careers, my uncle as a former Temptation and singer, and my aunt, Fay-Hauser Price, as an actress and producer. Their passion for storytelling and performance was uniquely intertwined with me and Jason's, which is why I named them our Hollywood parents. They were two true partners, in business and otherwise, and we were hopeful in our union, knowing that after years in the business of parenting, and love, we would still be as in love and intertwined as they were. I was grateful for their belief and trust in me.

My favorite and most heartwarming thought of them is the first Thanksgiving we spent together. It was their first time meeting me, and I was seven months pregnant. Though dinner was set for the early afternoon, we found ourselves cooking late into the evening. Our relationship was seamless and enjoyable.

The women on stage at the Waco Theatre were all dressed in black. Their presence was colorful, though most of them had the same brown skin. The diversity of actresses was mostly their intergenerational appeal. The presence of the piano on stage allowed me to create my own soundtrack, and its presence also served as an additional character. As each actress read a different monologue, I couldn't help but have flashbacks of what I've written. The title was "Listen to Her," and it was a letter to Taylor. I know over the years, I put her through changes of moving and new starts. I was in search of the good life. What I learned from my desperate pursuit is how the good life was not a destination but a lifelong journey. It's what you live every day when you open your eyes.

I've learned how the imperfections of life are what make us who we are. It builds us and molds us into better people; good people who want to do good things for other people. When the famous actress Marla Gibbs read the first line of my piece, I was transported back in time; the day I learned she was deaf in the nursery and the day I realized she would never hear my voice. Our bond and language have transcended time, and for years I would mouth, I love you. As I held my husband's hand, I was in awe of how out of 300 entries, mine was chosen. "I knew when I entered the hospital room she was deaf," she read. Giving voice to my experience as a mother and serving as one of the few monologues read that talked about a special-needs daughter. I named it "Listen to Her" for many reasons. During the season that I wrote "Listen to Her," I was also organizing a TEDx event by the same name. Ironically months before, the #MeToo Movement unleashed a truth which was dormant for years: it's time to listen to women.

Three months prior, I stood on a stage for a TEDx Talk while eight months pregnant and told my story. After learning at birth that my daughter had special needs, I raised her on my own while obtaining three academic degrees, including one from Yale. Despite our circumstances, we were able to live a good life. Now, I'm married and achieving different milestones. Giving a TEDx talk—and telling my story—was perhaps one of the most important events of my life yet.

The stage was set. I'd worked tirelessly on my speech and planned every detail meticulously. My goal was to impact others with my story and encourage the audience to consider that parents of children with special needs also want a good personal life. In order to assure that I had footage from the event, I hired an amazing production team: Natalie Perez, a talented videographer; and Rhasaan Nichols, a filmmaker and fellow Yalie.

But something went wrong.

As the backstage crew prepped the audio equipment; they seemed unsure about the quality of the sound. As they scrambled for clarity and guidance, I called Natalie to come backstage. She offered the production team her experienced advice. She also offered to film the entire event. They declined.

They did not listen to her guidance at all.

What happened next seemed surreal. As I gave my seven-minute talk, I was barely being heard by the audience. The audio was bad. It was so unclear that I paused mid-speech to do a mic check.

"Hold on audience, can you hear me?"

Did they hear me? Were they hearing my passion? Were they hearing my hard work? All I could do during the speech to keep up my confidence was convince myself that they had heard me. After the speech ended, I walked off the stage and was greeted by the TEDx staff. It must have been bad, because the staff member who greeted me had tears in his eyes.

I took off my heels and met my production person, Rhasaan. He was also upset but able to remain somewhat calm as he told me the audience not only heard my voice but also the voices of the backstage crew. Because of the technical difficulties, the audience was not given the opportunity to listen.

As I remained composed, I was met by my mentor, Lorri, and my videographer. It is imperative that women support women. At that moment I needed them, and they were there for me. They also remained composed but instructed me to do my entire speech again. My videographer was adamant. She insisted that I tell the organizers to allow me to redo my talk during intermission.

Though I could have had reasons to resist—excuses and fear—I listened to her.

There are countless occasions when women are not listened to. It happens at work, in the checkout line, and especially in male-centric settings where we are outnumbered. There is no price to the act of listening. However, there is a price—sometimes heftier that the perpetrators are willing to pay—when they do not listen. It is a high cost for everyone involved to ignore the women in the room.

Listening to women does not mean that you automatically do what they suggest, but it does mean that you take the time to consider their recommendations and suggestions. So much time, energy, and credibility could have been saved if someone had listened to our production team.

During the intermission, I performed my talk again. Ironically, in the green room, I received advice from a prominent businessman Winn Claybaugh, the dean and co-owner of Paul Mitchell Schools. Because I was eight months pregnant and had been in my heels all day, he told me to wear my sneakers.

I listened to him.

My second take of the speech went well, and my production team SheTv Media filmed and produced the video. It is the only official footage from the event.

Listen to women. We have so much to say and so much to contribute.

CPSIA information can be obtained
at www.ICGtesting.com
Printed in the USA
LVHW090748230420
653648LV00001BA/1/J